Praise for
LIFEPOINTS

"I like *LifePoints*. It provides a great new way to achieve weight control without sacrificing the nutritional quality of your diet. I'm sure it can make a real difference to the lives of millions of Americans."

—R. GAURTH HANSEN, PH.D., *Professor of Nutrition and Biochemistry, Utah State University*

"*LifePoints* is an elegantly simple and extremely practical guide based on sound scientific principles. It will help you make nutritional choices that will revolutionize your health."

—NEAL D. BARNARD, M.D., *Professor, Institute for Disease Prevention, George Washington University, President, Physician's Committee for Responsible Medicine*

"Dietary change toward a healthier life-style is scientifically justifiable and essential for our future. The *LifePoints* program makes that change as easy as any program available."

—T. COLIN CAMPBELL, PH.D., *Jacob Gould Schurman Professor of Nutritional Biochemistry, Cornell University*

"*LifePoints* is a valuable resource for those who wish to improve their health through diet and exercise. Adherence to the principles in this book may reduce the cancer rate and save lives."

—MICHAEL OSBORN, M.D. MS FRCS FACS, *President, Strang Cancer Prevention Center, affiliated with the New York Hospital—Cornell Medical Center*

"Having a long-term interest in helping individuals eat wisely, I am encouraged by and enthusiastic about the *Life-Points* system. *LifePoints* will be very useful to the consumer who wants to make wise eating decisions based on current research. It simplifies the abstract and complicated concept of nutritional quality. Very best wishes to you in all of your efforts."

—BONITA W. WYSE, *Dean, College of Family Life, Professor, Department of Nutrition and Food Sciences Utah State University*

"LifePoints provides solutions to the complex dietary decisions we face in the 1990s and beyond. It makes healthful eating an easily achieved goal for us all."

—DAVID PERLMUTTER, M.D., *President, Perlmutter Health Center, Author of "LifeGuide— Your Guide to a Longer and Healthier Life"*

"Putting dietary recommendations into practice can be a challenge. *LifePoints* is a user-friendly, practical approach to meal planning that helps take the guesswork out of what to eat for dinner tonight. It's a good-sense system that cuts the confusion as it guides you to a healthy eating style."

—SUZANNE HAVALA, MS, RD, *Charter Fellow of the American Dietetic Association*

"This book represents an important step in improving healthy nutritional compliance for our children in an era of excessive media hype and contradictory scientific studies."

—DAVID T. NASH, M.D., *Clinical Professor of Medicine, State University of New York, Health Science Center at Syracuse*

"LifePoints is the simplest system available for translating sound nutritional science into good dietary habits. All you have to do is use it."

—OLIVER ALABASTER, M.D., *Professor of Medicine, George Washington University, Director, Institute for Disease Prevention George Washington University Medical Center*

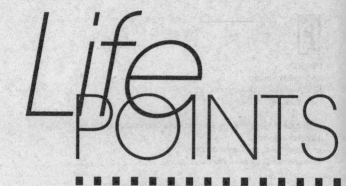

Life POINTS

Peter Cox &
Peggy Brusseau

A FIRESIDE BOOK
Published by Simon & Schuster

FIRESIDE
Rockefeller Center
1230 Avenue of the Americas
New York, NY 10020

The 1995 edition was first published in Great Britain by
Bloomsbury Publishing Plc.

FIRESIDE and colophon are registered trademarks
of Simon & Schuster Inc.

Designed by Irving Perkins Associates, Inc.

Manufactured in the United States of America

10 9 8 7 6 5 4 3 2 1

Library of Congress Cataloging-in-Publication Data
Cox, Peter.
   Lifepoints : the diet to count on / Peter Cox & Peggy Brusseau.
      p.   cm.
   1. Reducing diets.   I. Brusseau, Peggy.   II. Title.
RM222.2.C655   1997
613.2'5—dc21   97-13141   CIP
ISBN 0-684-83373-5

PUBLISHER'S NOTE

We would like to dedicate this book to our two wonderful children, Louis and Beau, who patiently understood while their parents toiled long hours over a hot word processor; also, to every kind person—and there are a great many—who helped us discover, refine, and improve the LifePoints system in some way. Readers, scientists, publishers, friends, and supporters —*LifePoints* simply would not exist without you!

CONTENTS ....

STOP! DON'T TURN
ANOTHER PAGE ....

• First let us show you just how easy it is to use the revolutionary new LifePoints system. We believe that LifePoints is the most powerful food control system in the world—but what really counts is what *you* think of it. Here's your chance to road-test the system, in less than sixty seconds!

First: Turn to the LifePoints Counter starting on page 125 and flip through all the foods until you find a couple of alternative items that you *might* want to eat at your next meal. Quick example: For breakfast, you might eat a croissant, or you might choose to have a bagel. For your convenience, the foods are listed in similar groups (e.g. "Breads") but if you can't quickly find what you're looking for, just use the Index at the very end of the book.

Next:	Now, check out the RiskPoints and Life-Points numbers for both foods (croissant/bagel). At this juncture, all you need to know is that the RiskPoints number tells you how much *bad stuff* there is in the food you're looking at, and the LifePoints number tells you how much *good stuff* it contains. Simple, isn't it?
Finally:	Just aim to keep your RiskPoints intake *low* and your LifePoints intake *high*. Following our example: A butter croissant has 50 Risk-Points, but the bagel only has 2, so immediately you can tell that the bagel is likely to be a better bet. Now look at the LifePoints number: croissant 6, bagel 8. The bagel wins in both categories! *Voilà!*

Congratulations—you've just completed the Life-Points Lift-off, and you've just proved to yourself how phenomenally easy it is to use the LifePoints system. But that was just a single example. You can actually use LifePoints to accomplish much, much more, as you'll find out in the following pages. No matter what your individual food tastes are, or what kind of eating style you prefer, LifePoints will work *with* you and *for* you.

First, LifePoints affords us an effective way of controlling and then maintaining weight—something that is both easier and more effective than calorie-counting or any other nine-days' diet wonder. Second, it lets you know that for every mouthful you eat, you are getting maximum nutritional health benefits. And third, LifePoints is a friendly system that *empowers* you to make the right choices, but doesn't *enslave* you by making you feel guilty—because, hey, food is one of life's great pleasures!

If you agree with us that these three things are important to you, then we know that you're going to like LifePoints.

Peter & Peggy

INTRODUCTION: MEET YOUR FOOD TOOL ....

• How on earth did the human race ever manage to survive before there were diet books?

Pardon our cynicism. We recently checked the "Books In Print" database and found to our astonishment that there are more than five thousand different diet books available to the American public. If you read one every day, it would take you over thirteen years to digest them!

So, does the world really *need* one more diet book? Probably not, but then, *LifePoints* isn't just another diet book that follows the invariable "buy it, trash it" formula. You see, *LifePoints* isn't trying to sell you an impossible dream. It doesn't promise you thin thighs in thirty days; it's not selling you a mind-changing philosophy; nor does it make outlandish claims for the latest "miracle breakthrough" food supplement, pill, or potion. In fact, *LifePoints* isn't selling you anything.

So what is *LifePoints?* It is a tool. It is said that knowledge is power. If that is so, then you have in your hands one of the most powerful tools for personal health that you are ever likely to find. When you think about it, we have tools to help us in almost every area of our lives: labor-saving tools around the home, software tools to aid in gathering and interpreting data, learning tools to educate ourselves and our children. But when it comes to managing the food we eat, most of us are thoroughly shortchanged. What effective tools do we *really* have? Over five thousand diet books, that's what—each one with a different sales pitch! Five thousand different and often conflicting sets of advice on achieving dietary nirvana. Not likely.

Thanks to all those diet books, each promising unrealistic gains if only you will agree to restrict your eating to just what they tell you to eat, we have become a society that now interprets the very word *diet* to mean "weight loss regime." What a grossly inaccurate perversion of meaning that is! As if the only point of eating (or in the case of diet books, not eating) is to try to lose weight. On the contrary, we believe that your expectations for your "diet" should be far higher than that. Indeed, this is what we believe your "diet" should do for you:

- It should provide you with an optimum intake of all the life-protecting, health-enhancing nutrients that nature gives us.

- It should steer you away from dangerous, unhealthy, or unwholesome foods that imperil your health (obesity is one, but only one, result of an unhealthy diet).
- And—yes!—it should be fun, tasty, and so satisfying that it leaves you feeling contented and well-nourished.

For decades, diet books have operated on the premise that you must effectively relinquish power of attorney over your life. That's the second-rate deal they're offering: "Do what I tell you, and in return you'll lose weight." We find that attitude unacceptable, disrespectful to the reader, and highly manipulative. You see, they have to manipulate you as part of the process whereby they hype you about the diet, thus building your expectations and motivation, but when you fail (and failure is all but inevitable, sooner or later, because dieting can only work in the short term), they make you feel responsible: *You* were not good enough; *you* didn't pass muster; *you* failed again. Feel the guilt!

We do not believe that people fail diets. On the contrary, it's the diet that usually fails the person. The LifePoints system doesn't rely on guilt to motivate and it will never boss you around. Because LifePoints doesn't operate on a win/lose paradigm, it is actually impossible for you to "fail." Unlike conventional diets, there's no such thing as staying on or falling off the LifePoints system. Every time you use LifePoints, you benefit. That's right—every time. If you've experimented with LifePoints Lift-off, you've already discovered just how easy the system really is. The LifePoints learning curve is smooth and gradual, and most important, you'll discover that LifePoints does not "lock you in." LifePoints is a real-world, practical food tool, just like all the other tools you use every day, in all other aspects of your life.

Our goal in creating the LifePoints concept was to devise a way to measure the good things, and bad things, in our foods and to put that information right at your fingertips so that you can have an effective road map in deciding what to eat.

Early on in our research, we encountered the same sort of cynicism that colors most diet books. Naysayers told us that what we intended to do was either impossible, or worse, not worth doing. The latter revealed a depth of cynicism that quite frankly appalled us. These experts and health professionals actually admitted when pressed that yes, they were prescribing diets for their patients that were too high in fats and other undesirable foodstuffs, but they went on to explain it was necessary to do so "because our patients won't eat anything better."

We disagree. Apparently we have more faith in our readers than the experts had in their own patients. We believe that most people would be delighted to eat "better" provided that they were given a method of planning for themselves. The idea behind LifePoints was not to prescribe yet another rigid diet but to create a flexible and simple tool for people to use creatively, as they wished. And we believe our instincts were right, because the bottom line is this: Ordering someone to follow a rigid, predetermined diet is almost always a recipe for failure. But give people tools with which to plan their own diet, and they will almost always succeed.

Every year an estimated 80 million Americans go on a diet, but no matter how much weight they lose, 95 percent of those people gain it back, which is excellent news for America's $50 billion diet industry, because it ensures a steady flow of repeat business— but for the individual dieters who comprise that dismal statistic, it's an unmitigated disaster. The real scandal of the diet industry is that it turns people away from a healthy relationship with their food. And who can blame them? If your umpteenth diet has failed miserably, once again, then drifting into obesity does seem the only option left. If you factor into this equation the powerful role played by today's fast-food junk-food behemoth (the Agriculture Department estimates they spend $36 billion a year on advertising alone!) and consider how we are constantly besieged with messages urging us to binge, binge, binge, then you begin to appreciate what the average dieter is up against.

Food, in case you hadn't realized, is a very political issue, and the hearts and minds—not to mention the stomachs—of consumers are at the very center of the battle. Every day there seems to be a new controversy, with contradictory reports in the headlines about food. If you want to avoid heart disease, cut your cholesterol. If you want to avoid cancer, *don't* cut your cholesterol. Eat lots of fruit to get a high antioxidant intake. Eat lots of fruit, and you'll get pesticide poisoning. We've all seen hundreds of stories like these and most of us have become more and more confused by them.

Pick up virtually any food in the supermarket today, and you'll be bombarded with nutritional food information on the label. Increasingly, food manufacturers are displaying more and more of such information on their products—indeed, the rules and regulations seem to grow more complex and demanding each year. But here's the strange paradox: While there's never been so much information available to the consumer, it's *never* been more difficult to understand what it all means! We'd bet that not one consumer in a million actually uses all this data. And that is not surprising. Just consider some of the insurmountable obstacles you'd face: Nutritional information on food labels is often presented as the amount of vitamins or minerals present in 100 grams of the food. But people don't eat in neat, 100-gram servings! Just working out the calories in a serving is difficult enough, but have you ever tried adding up all the vitamins and minerals? Don't—unless you want to carry a portable computer around with you. If you want a quick migraine, try solving this: Food A has 0.6 milligrams of niacin in a serving, and 72 milligrams of vitamin C. Food B has 1.2 milligrams of niacin per serving, and 5 milligrams of vitamin C. Now: Work out which is the most nutritious food to buy—and good luck! We'll check with you in the next century.

These problems are just the tip of a Titanic-sized iceberg. While appearing to give us increased nutritional information, today's food labels too often deprive us of effective control over the food we eat. Too much information—especially if it's nearly impossible to use—is just as bad as too little information. The purpose of LifePoints is to enable readers to see the forest through the trees. Consumers shouldn't have to become scientists in order to get the big picture, and that's what LifePoints gives you. We did the scientific homework to create the algorithm necessary to decipher the big picture, which is what all of us really want to know. Because LifePoints presents the reader with enough information to make effective decisions, but not so much that you're drowning in data, it effectively gives you control over your food intake. In a word, it *empowers* you.

LifePoints takes the philosophy of empowerment —now proven to be very effective—to its ultimate conclusion. Quite simply, LifePoints is the world's first easy-to-use guide to the goodness in food. It lets you compare one food with another and see which is better for you. It lets you scrutinize your present diet, and correct it if necessary. It lets you plan a permanently healthy way of eating, and lets you change it whenever you want to. And these are things that no book has ever done before.

When you buy a book, you naturally want to know a few things about the people who wrote it, and their reasons for doing so. Peggy is American, and Peter is British. We're married with two children, and divide our time between the two countries. We've written about food and health for about ten years, but we're not doctors. We wrote this book because we became increasingly dismayed by the mounting confusion that exists about our diets and health.

Today, virtually every common disease can either be prevented or considerably alleviated by dietary means. The latest figures reveal that chronic illnesses now affect about 100 million Americans—four in every ten people—and cost the nation about $425 billion a year for health care expenses. These people are not disabled, but live with the threat of relapses that could result in lost work days, hospitalization, and higher health costs. They account for about 80 percent of all hospital stays.

Yet for decades, the world's medical and scientific journals have published thousands upon thousands of epidemiological studies and intervention studies that give us a unique insight into the health benefits of particular patterns of eating, individual foodstuffs, and indeed specific nutrients. Unbelievably, this for-midable body of knowledge rarely escapes the nar-row confines of academia to move into the wider world. That this desperately needed information re-mains largely unknown by the general public is a very serious indictment of the way that science is permitted to function in the real world. Our skill is to take the vital results that science can generate and translate them into plain language and a plan of action that ordinary people such as ourselves can actually use right now.

In many diet books authors choose to dress themselves up with impressive-sounding qualifications, degrees, and doctorates. We've never felt the need to pretend to be anything other than what we are—first and foremost, LifePoints users, the couple behind the checkout line, people who have more in common with their readers than with the white coat community. After all, LifePoints succeeds or fails on the basis of how well it actually works for you. Even so, we've been very fortunate to garner endorsements for Life-Points from a number of the nation's most distinguished scientists and researchers, to whom we express our most sincere gratitude.

When LifePoints was first published in Britain (whose national diet is, if anything, less healthy than the American one) it attracted some highly flattering media coverage, including that of Britain's most popular quality national newspaper, the *Daily Mail*, who simply wrote: "LifePoints is the diet revolution of the decade." Everyone knows it's bad to believe your press, but we honestly do believe that LifePoints represents a quantum leap forward in healthy eating. We can promise you that once you've used the LifePoints system for just a few days, it will permanently change the way you think about food. For the first time ever, LifePoints gives you the big picture about the healthy and unhealthy aspects of your food intake. If knowledge is power, then you've just taken the first step toward power over your diet—forever!

Part One ·························

THE LIFEPOINTS REVOLUTION

• When you think about food you've been conditioned to think about calories. A fresh apple has about 80 calories. A serving of baked beans has about 300. A cheeseburger, about 600. That's how we've been trained to measure the value of the food we eat.

But calories are by no means a satisfactory gauge of a food's worth or importance to the human body and its well-being. What judgment can you truly make about a food that yields, say, 300 calories? Can you tell whether that food is *good* for you, or *bad* for you? Is it a healthy food or a health hazard? Will it tend to fortify or weaken your state of health? How well does it fit into the rest of your day's diet? Is it going to make you put on fat or lose weight? Does it contain health-enhancing nutrients or disease-promoting anti-nutrients?

Just knowing a food's calorie yield cannot possibly answer any of these vital questions. And yet, that's the only basis by which most of us have ever tried to assess the quality of the food we consume.

And what the heck is a "calorie" anyway? You may be surprised to find out. Unlike other nutrients in food, you can't isolate calories. Give an orange to a biochemist, and after some chemical manipulation in the lab, she'll be able to give you a test tube with most of that orange's vitamin C neatly separated out. Similarly with most other nutrients. But not calories. That's because calories have no tangible existence on their own. You can't see them, you can't taste them, and you certainly can't separate them out from the food itself. In Latin, "calor" means "heat," and that gives us a clue to the real role of the calorie. It is simply the name of a unit used to measure heat energy.

One calorie was originally defined as the amount of heat energy required to raise the temperature of one gram of water one degree Centigrade—from 14.5°C. to 15.5°C. Pretty obscure, isn't it? Today, a calorie is defined in mechanical rather than thermal terms, so that one calorie equals 4.184 watt-seconds (or joules). Like feet, inches, meters, pints, and liters, the calorie unit is a useful measure when used properly. For example, it takes 80 calories to melt one gram of ice. It takes 540 calories to boil one gram of water. Burn one gram of carbon and you'll release 7,830 calories. Run vigorously and you'll expend about 15,000 calories a minute (yes, fifteen *thousand*

—if you find this a bit puzzling, read on!). All interesting enough, but what does it tell us about the quality of our food?

Not much!

Merely knowing the amount of heat energy locked up inside the food we eat isn't going to tell us much about that food's quality, or its impact on our health. Scientists have conventionally used something called a "bomb calorimeter" to measure the calorie yield of a food. They take a portion of the food in question— say a slice of cheesecake—and seal it inside a container. The air is pumped out and pure oxygen is pumped in. Then, an electric spark ignites the oxygen and—kaboom!—the food burns, and heat energy is released. The container is immersed in a water bath, and by measuring the rise in the water's temperature it is possible to calculate the calorie yield of the food. Now does that sound *anything like* what goes on in your stomach? We hope not.

In fact, this standard laboratory technique is imperfect. Not all the energy locked up in food is available to the human metabolic processes. Although humans have an astoundingly large surface area of digestive tract through which the nutrients in foods are absorbed (if you spread it out it would be larger than a tennis court), we don't absorb *all* the nutrients in food, and we don't use *all* the potential heat energy locked up in foodstuffs. Real world systems, such as digestion, are always far more complex than laboratory models.

The calorie yield of a food, as approximated by

the bomb calorimeter, tells us something about the amount of heat energy locked up inside a food, but nothing more. And by the way, just to complicate matters, a "calorie" when used in connection with food usually means a "kilocalorie," or 1000 calories. Sometimes you'll see it written "kcal," and sometimes "Cal." From now onward in this book, we're going to follow the normal, although rather illogical, convention of saying "calorie" when we really mean "kilocalorie." Well, no one ever claimed that nutrition was a perfect science.

So here you are, planning your diet. You're looking at food labels in the supermarket, and all you can really do is compare the calorie yield of one food with another. You pick up two cans, and both labels show approximately the same calorie yield. Which one are you going to choose? With only one nutritional dimension to work with, you might as well flip a coin. And what's even more disturbing is an awkard little fact that's received surprisingly little publicity: Food labels are often wrong! When scientists checked the *actual* calorie yield of foods (as measured by the bomb calorimeter) and compared it to the *stated* calorie yield on the label, they got a big surprise.[1]

Take another scenario. You've decided to get serious about this calorie-counting business, so you've bought a calorie counter. Let's say you've decided to limit yourself to about 1800 calories a day. So you diligently plan your day's food intake, calculator in hand, pencil and eraser at the ready, and holy mackerel, is it hard work! Juggling all those portion sizes, searching for a food that you can just squeeze into the limit—and, let's face it, doing a bit of cheating, too. Finally, you've done it—1800 calories, or thereabouts. But what have you *really* achieved? Have you assured yourself a good intake of all the essential vitamins? Probably not. Have you made sure that your day's food intake is healthily low in fat? Maybe. Have you achieved *anything at all* other than keeping your energy intake down to 1800 calories? You're probably not sure.

Here's the bottom line. Calories are merely a one-dimensional measure of a food's worth. They can tell you about its energy yield, and no more. *Using calories—and only calories—to plan a healthy diet is about as sensible as trying to drive down a crowded highway with one eye shut.*

You're simply not getting enough information to do the job properly.

If the Only Tool You Have Is a Hammer, All Problems Begin To Look Like Nails

It's not hard to understand why calories have loomed so large in our food consciousness in recent decades. The only dietary sources of calories are carbohydrates, proteins, fats, and alcohol. If your combined caloric intake of these substances greatly exceeds the amount of energy you expend, then your body very sensibly stores the excess energy as fat. We say "very sensibly" because this marvelous ability to store food energy efficiently is one of our most impressive biological characteristics. We should be proud of the fact that humans are one of the most successful species ever to walk, swim, or crawl over the surface of planet earth, and our phenomenally efficient energy storage system is surely one of the most important factors in our success. Did you know that we have more fat cells (called adipocytes) in proportion to our body mass than virtually *any other creature*—only hedgehogs and whales have a greater proportion of fat cells in their bodies. Even animals that we traditionally think of as "fatties," such as pigs, seals, bears, and camels, all have proportionately fewer fat cells than we do! Far from being a curse, this high proportion of fat cells is actually a tremendous evolutionary advantage, because it allows us to cope with the uncertainty of a variable food supply—we can smooth out the peaks and troughs. No food today? No problem! We can live off our fat!

Of course, most Americans don't have that particular problem any more. For most of us, there are *no* days without food, only days when there's too much, far too easily available. And that's one big reason why 33.4 percent of Americans aged twenty years or older are overweight.[2] What was once a major biological advantage has suddenly and treacherously turned into a life-threatening problem. Today, humans are the only animal species to be so seriously menaced by obesity.

And let's face facts. In general, people put on excess baggage because they eat inappropriately. The truth is, you either control your food or it controls you. Yes, other factors are sometimes involved in the development of obesity, such as our genetic predisposition, what our mothers ate before and during pregnancy, and whether or not we were breast-fed when young. But none of these factors should be allowed to obscure this central, most vital truth: Most of us are not in control of the food we eat. A recent experiment at St. Luke's-Roosevelt Hospital Center in New York demonstrated this very convincingly.[3]

They took a group of people who had been labeled "diet-resistant"—chronic dieting failures who had never lost weight, even though they claimed to have been on regimes as low as 1200 calories a day. The doctors measured all the calories these people took in and burned up, and found that their metabolisms were *perfectly normal*—there was no genetic defect, no overactive thyroid, no exotic metabolic problem. No. The real problem was quite clear: They were simply eating too much! And they were fooling themselves about how much they ate—they were actually taking in *twice as many* calories as they thought they were. To make matters worse, they were actually taking about half as much exercise as they believed they were getting, too. A clear-cut case of self-deception. Commented Dr. Steven B. Heymsfield, head of the weight control unit at the hospital: "These people really cannot invoke some genetic cause as the only explanation for their obesity. The main reason they are overweight is that they are overeating. Let's not blame it on something that it isn't."[4] That's telling it like it is. Tempting though it may be to blame our rapidly increasing girth on "bad genes," that explanation simply doesn't pass the acid test. As another scientist, Dr. George Bray, editor of the journal *Obesity Research,* points out: "Our genes haven't changed in the past ten years."[5]

. . . .
TIP: Never go to the supermarket hungry! People who shop on full stomachs can more easily resist those impulse buys of high-fat, low-nutrition food.
. . . .

For some people, the prospect of being able to shift the blame for their weight problem to "bad genes" is heartening, because it conveniently excuses them from any responsibility in the matter of their spreading waistline. However, we take the opposite approach. Clearly, all of us have the potential to learn to choose what we should eat, and when we should eat it. Just because most of us aren't very good at taking control over our food intake (and why should we be when most of us have never been taught how to?) doesn't mean that we have to find a scapegoat to blame for the inevitable consequences that follow from eating a poor diet. Instead of excuses, let's use this precious opportunity to learn how to reclaim this vital area of our lives!

So *why* do we overeat? Here, we can be much kinder to ourselves. In the main, the cause of overeating isn't gluttony, greed, or some character failing. Actually, it's biology. Once again, it's all to do with our species' ancient (and until recently) highly successful feeding strategy. Animals in their natural environment *never* die from overeating; the greater threat comes, of course, from starvation. In nature, the best survival strategy is to eat whenever you get the opportunity, because you never know where your next meal's coming from. That's why many of us still eat whenever we get the chance, even though logic tells us that there is no conceivable likelihood of the average American starving to death. Today, inside our twenty-first century minds and bodies, there are the genetic remnants of our ancestral heritage from many millennia ago. The appendix, the coccyx (tail bone), the webbing that still exists between our fingers—these and other physical clues indicate that our prehuman ancestry is still very much a part of our makeup. Although our human ancestors split from the ancestors of chimpanzees all of seven million years ago, there is only the smallest (about 1.6 percent) genetic difference between modern humans and chimpanzees, which shows you just how slowly evolution takes place. And that's really at the root of most of our dietary problems.

S. Boyd Eaton, Marjorie Shostak, and Melvin Konner are three scientists whose work has done much to enable us to understand the causes of the dietary problems we all face today. "Here we are," they note, "in the late twentieth century, with a forty-thousand-year-old model body . . . adjusting as best we can to the complex demands of our lives. Yet with genetic makeups essentially out of sync with our life-styles, an inevitable discordance exists between the world we live in today and the world our genes 'think' we live in still. This mismatch . . . can account for many of our ills, especially the 'chronic diseases of civilization' that cause 75 percent of the deaths in industrial societies."[6]

These same scientists have clearly shown that the "Stone Age" diet we are genetically programmed to consume differs in some vitally important ways from the type of diet most of us consume today. Some of the key differences are shown in Charts One, Two, and Three. You'll be pleased to know that the Life-Points system incorporates many features of the Stone Age diet. More about this later.

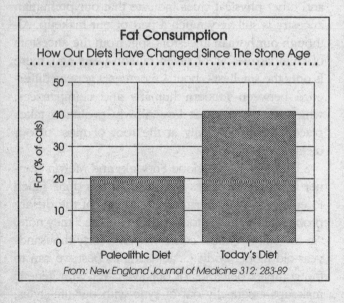

Fat Consumption
How Our Diets Have Changed Since The Stone Age

From: *New England Journal of Medicine 312: 283-89*

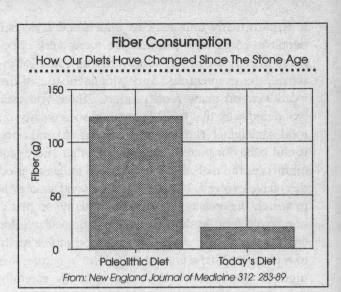

Fiber Consumption

How Our Diets Have Changed Since The Stone Age

From: New England Journal of Medicine 312: 283-89

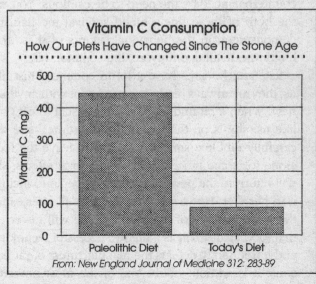

Vitamin C Consumption

How Our Diets Have Changed Since The Stone Age

From: New England Journal of Medicine 312: 283-89

It is particularly important to understand how our deep-rooted survival instincts are today very effectively manipulated by food advertising. Take, for instance, the frequent and very prominent use of the word *new* on many food products. Have you ever wondered why this word is featured so regularly on food packaging? The answer lies in an old and once useful behavior pattern that we and other successful omnivores (animals that have adapted to eat a varied diet) have evolved. The successful survival strategy is to search out *new* types of food regularly, so that if one staple food in the diet becomes unavailable for any reason, there is always another food source ready to replace it. What a great strategy! But in nature, this urge to experiment with new food is carefully counterbalanced by the need to be cautious. You can see both of these finely tuned survival mechanisms demonstrated in the behavior patterns of that other hugely flourishing omnivore, the common rat.

Rats and humans have a lot in common. Just like us, they are always ready to experiment with anything new. When a rat finds something unusual to eat (and like us, she is on the lookout all the time), she will carefully nibble a small amount, then leave the food alone for some time. If she suffers no ill effects, she will return to the new food and may begin to include it in her diet. However, if the rat feels ill after eating that small sample of "new" food, she will never eat that food again. This is a highly successful technique, and it frequently defeats the manufacturers of rat poisons. It is without doubt one of the most powerful feeding strategies of all time, because it reconciles two opposing imperatives:

- The ceaseless quest to find new food sources
- The urge to be cautious when faced with unknown danger

We humans use precisely the same technique. You can prove it for yourself: Think back to a time when you felt ill soon after eating a particular type of food. It doesn't really matter whether your sickness was actually caused by the food you remember eating. What matters is that you now associate that food with the unpleasant feelings afterward, and in all probability, you will never eat that particular food again.

It's in these ways that our old survival mechanisms try to keep us away from foods that may be dangerous for us. However, it's the other side of this mechanism —the strong instinct we all possess to experiment with anything "new"—that gets us into so much trouble these days, simply because there's *so much* temptation all around us. It is this constant desire to look for—and experiment with—new foodstuffs that makes us so vulnerable to overeating.

With these immensely powerful instincts tempting us to eat whenever we can and try that new food right now, it's hardly surprising that, in today's world of promiscuous consumption, many of us eat far too much. It's not that we're weak-willed. It's just that *we can't fight nature*.

Once you begin to understand this, you'll appreciate why, in truth, we really don't have a calorie problem. Actually, we have something far more serious—a food strategy problem.

The proof is all around us. Scientific data show that the American male body mass index (a measure of obesity) has increased by 16 percent over the last century, in line with increasing affluence and the ever-increasing availability of new, cheap, and often unhealthy foodstuffs. Here's a rather more trivial but equally telling example: When New York's Yankee Stadium was built in 1922, the width of each seat was set to a generous nineteen inches. Fifty years later, the average American posterior had broadened so much that the seats had to be widened to twenty-two inches. After thirty years of applied research into obesity, and a public expenditure of more than $100 billion in America alone, people are fatter than ever before!

Let's be quite clear about this. Calling obesity a "calorie problem" is about as sensible as calling alcoholism a "cup problem." In both cases, the units of measurement are being confused with the real issue. There's an old saying that goes: "If the only tool you have is a hammer, all problems begin to look like nails." We could update that to say: "If the only tool you have is a calorie counter, every dietary problem begins to look like a calorie problem."

And here's why it really matters so very much: As long as we interpret obesity to be caused by an excess of calories, the treatment for obesity will simply be to reverse the process, by trying to consume fewer calories. That process is called "going on a diet."

But diets—as most of you know by now—simply don't work.

Diets! Who Needs Them?

When you drastically reduce your calorie intake, a number of serious things happen. First of all, your body thinks you're starving. As far as your body is concerned, dieting and starvation are one and the same thing. Your body has an excellent survival strategy built in, ready to be implemented at the drop of a calorie. The first thing it does is to lower your metabolism in order to conserve energy. The longer your food intake continues to be below what it expects, the harder your body tries to preserve that precious energy locked up as fat. That's why the first week of any calorie-restricted diet produces an impressive result, yet subsequent weeks achieve little, if anything. Your body's deep-rooted instincts are fighting you all the way. And sooner or later, they'll win. The survival of our species depended on it.

One particularly notorious way in which our instincts triumph over our willpower is through the binge impulse. You know the scenario: Your diet's lasted a few days, and so far it's gone well. Then, in one mad, unrestrained moment, you find yourself behaving like a great white shark in a popular swimming pool. Eat! Eat! Eat! As you manically bolt down everything in sight, you start to feel helpless and so very, very guilty. How *could* you be so weak? How *could* you have ruined all your hard work in a momentary feeding frenzy? This sort of negative self-talk can even lead to serious eating disorders such as bulimia. But take it easy on yourself for a moment. When you think about it, the binge impulse is, yet again, a very logical and successful feeding strategy. Your body thinks that there is a severe food shortage that is causing you to starve. Doing their best to protect you, your instincts become supersensitive to any potential source of food—and of course, in today's society there are unlimited sources of food available everywhere. Drop your guard for just one instant and those ancient survival instincts take over.

Also, dieting is a torture. You have to put up with absurdly small portion sizes of your favorite foods, and that requires superhuman discipline, or an unhealthy streak of masochism. Even worse, you feel hungry most of the time, which makes you a real pain in the you-know-what to your colleagues, friends, and family. Ever wonder why dieters have to club together in those self-help groups? Perhaps it's because nobody else wants to talk to them.

Joking aside, conventional calorie-restricted diets have even more serious drawbacks, too. Among the symptoms:

- Bloating and distended stomach
- Constipation

- Depression
- Failure to produce collagen, the major protein of all connective tissues
- Feeling cold all the time
- Hair loss
- Headaches
- Lack of energy
- Loss of lean tissue
- Low blood pressure leading to dizziness
- Menstrual difficulties
- Sleep disruption
- Water retention
- Yeast infections

There are enough scientific studies around now for us to come to the certain conclusion that dieting, as it's usually practiced, is ineffective in any long-term sense. In a 1988 Dutch study, men who experienced many stressful life events in a short period experienced a weight gain.[7] This is not unusual—once again, it's our body's way of trying to protect us from harm. A year later, this weight gain had disappeared in almost all subgroups of these men. The exception was the subgroup that tried to lose weight by dieting; those who dieted had gained yet more weight! This study, reported in the *International Journal of Obesity*, makes no sense to those who believe weight gain is a "calorie problem," and therefore weight loss can be accomplished simply by restricting calories. But when you see it in terms of a survival strategy, it makes perfect sense: Those men had already been through a number of stressful life events, and the threat posed by dieting (i.e. starvation) seemed, to their bodies, to be just one more hazard. Their survival mechanisms actually responded splendidly by trying to conserve every last calorie.

In fact, many scientific studies now confirm that if you want to put on weight, one of the very best ways to do it is to diet. Weight gain is particularly provoked by "diet cycling" (continual diet/binge cycles), and it is such a well-accepted phenomenon that it is sometimes used in a clinical situation to help underweight patients put on bulk. How, precisely, does this happen? It's probably connected to the production of an enzyme called lipoprotein lipase (LPL), which is responsible for storing body fat. When one starts a diet, LPL levels initially drop, then remorselessly rise again —sometimes to twenty-five times the normal level. The fatter you are to begin with, the more LPL you'll produce when dieting. This finding has been used to support the "set point" theory of body weight regulation, which suggests that each person has an internal control system that predetermines how much weight, or fat, we should have.

What it really boils down to is this: If calorie-restricted diets worked effectively, then there would be few people in the Western world with obesity problems. But in their seminal paper entitled "Diet and Health: Implications for Reducing Chronic Disease Risk," the Committee on Diet and Health of the National Research Council point out that "food intake has declined over the past decade when body weight and presumably fat stores have, on average, increased."[8] In other words, our growing fatness cannot be explained by the fact that we're consuming more calories, because we're not. Other studies have confirmed that Westerners today take in fewer calories than we did at the beginning of the twentieth century, yet the level of obesity has stubbornly climbed.

Let's sum up:

First: Merely knowing the heat yield of a foodstuff as measured in calories tells us next to nothing about its real nutritional worth to us.

Second: Conventional calorie-restricted diets have a very poor track record of success, and ultimately lead to weight gain more often than not.

Third: Since we're consuming fewer calories today than we used to, but are getting fatter, we can conclude that effective weight control must involve more than just counting calories.

As you'll see, the LifePoints approach toward effective weight control is the art of dieting without dieting. We don't believe that crash diets are effective in the long run, nor are they necessarily safe for you. Neither do we believe that strict calorie counting achieves any worthwhile change. Instead, the focus of the Life-Points system is to trust our bodies and instincts a little more, while providing a helping hand and a system for developing and reinforcing our instinctive wisdom about our food choices. The LifePoints system can help you to regularize your weight by directing you toward consciously eating good food and avoiding bad.

It's that simple, because that's how our basic human survival mechanism works.

So Many Experts; Whom Do You Trust?

The French statesman Charles de Gaulle once re-marked: "There are three certain ways to go to hell. The first is gambling, which is the quickest. The second is women, which is the most enjoyable. The third is believing experts, which is the most certain."

He might well have had the diet industry in mind with their legions of "experts." It's tragically ironic that there are so many dietary experts around, and yet millions of us still die every year from diet-related diseases. Actually, this excess of experts often only adds to the widespread chaos and confusion that exists today about healthy eating. Here's why:

- Science evolves through a dynamic process. One scientist proposes a theory; another scientist criticizes it. Yet another scientist weaves the elements together to make a new theory—and so the process continues. *But whose voice should you listen to?*

- You know, and we know, that some experts can be bought. If you look hard enough, you can find an expert to tell you almost anything you want to hear. For example, if you happen to manufacture the world's most unwholesome junk food and you want to find an expert to tell people that it's healthier than mother's milk, you'll eventually find one, *providing you're prepared to pay.* . . .

- The media's job is to bring us the latest news. And that's what it generally does. But when this week's diet fad turns into next week's diet nightmare, we don't always learn about it. *The next craze is already upon us.*

- Ultimately, all that most experts do is state their opinions, which may be right, wrong, or a bit of both. Opinions are cheap—everyone's got a whole bunch, and most of us are only too eager to give them away to anyone who'll listen! Opinions are also "predigested," by which we mean that they don't supply you with the knowledge or the understanding you need to form your own views. Fundamentally, most experts are really saying, "Take my word for it." *Why should we?*

Furthermore, the fragmentary nature of the information we receive from the media today is deeply disturbing. We monitored the news over a few weeks, and came up with the following stories:

- Alfalfa lowers cholesterol!
- Celery lowers blood pressure!
- Kudzu root can cure alcoholism!
- Garlic's antioxidants can fight cancer!
- Avocados lower cholesterol [yes, really]!
- Phenols in red wine prevent heart disease!
- Flavonoids in fruit can prevent heart disease!
- Genistein in soya products blocks tumor growth!
- Chinese bitter melon can fight viruses including HIV!
- Broccoli fights breast cancer by boosting anticancer enzymes!

These are typical of the kind of news stories we are all continually exposed to. In each case, there is credible scientific evidence to support the claim being made. But, realistically, how can you actually *use* these news items? Should you try to eat a diet based on alfalfa, broccoli, celery, garlic, and red wine? Doesn't that sound rather, well—deranged?

And that's the problem. If you try to plan a healthy diet using nothing but scraps of information like these, you'll certainly fail, and probably go half-crazy in the process. The truth is that stories such as these have very little practical use. Yes, they're interesting to read about. But can you put the information to good use? No!

That's why LifePoints takes exactly the opposite approach. We're interested first and foremost in showing you the *big picture*. By applying decades of human population studies, we've built up a clear image of the major healthy and unhealthy factors in the human diet. For example, the evidence is convincing that people who consume significant quantities of saturated fat have a high incidence of heart disease, so saturated fat is obviously a major risk factor in our diets. On the other hand, people who eat foods that are high in the antioxidant beta-carotene have much less heart disease and fewer cancers, which indicates that beta-carotene is one of the important health-protectors. Many of these nutritional factors will already be familiar to you (all of them are described in the following pages). However, *never before* have you had the opportunity to see how they all add up to make a healthy or unhealthy food. Now, you can.

In developing the LifePoints system, one of the most powerful tools we have used is a relatively new science called epidemiology. As the name suggests, it evolved from the scientific study of epidemics. In 1854, a scientist called John Snow investigated and described an epidemic of cholera in London, which —by careful scientific detective work—he found had originated from one contaminated water well. He is generally recognized as the first epidemiologist of the modern era. Now, the most important point about Snow's work, and about most epidemiology, is this: He traced the cholera outbreak back to contaminated drinking water *many years before* the bacillus that causes cholera was finally discovered and identified. More recently, epidemiologic studies have resulted in detailed descriptions of hepatitis, Lassa fever, Legionnaires' disease, and toxic shock syndrome far in advance of the identification of their causative agents. Also, the connection between smoking and lung cancer was first made from epidemiologic studies—again, well before laboratory experiments finally established the cause-and-effect relationship. Because it concentrates on studying the way things *actually work* in the real world, rather than the way laboratory scientists might like them to be, epidemiology is capable of giving us remarkably early warning signals.

Epidemiology can tell us a lot about good diets and bad diets, and about good foods and bad foods. When you look at all the different dietary customs, fashions, tastes, and habits of the world's population, you discover some surprising things. Take a look at the chart on page 51, which compares the diets of three very different countries—the United States (a typical Western diet), Greece (a typical Mediterranean one), and Japan (a typical Far Eastern one). You can see that in almost every area, the three countries have quite different dietary tastes. For example, meat consumption is very high in the U.S., and low in the other two. Saturated fat consumption is high in the U.S. (18 percent of all calories consumed are from saturated fat), half that in Greece (8 percent of all calories), and very low indeed in Japan (3 percent). One of the greatest strengths of epidemiology lies in its ability to observe how diets change over time (for example, both red meat and saturated fat consumption are currently increasing rapidly in both Greece and Japan) and relate these shifts to the changing patterns of disease and causes of death. This is one clear and

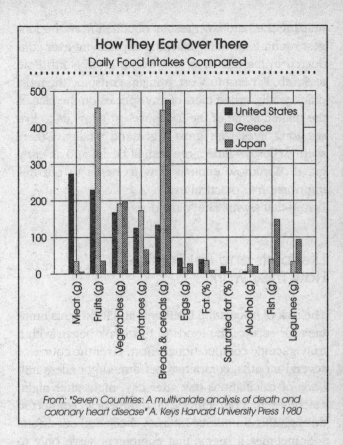

How They Eat Over There
Daily Food Intakes Compared

Legend:
- United States
- Greece
- Japan

Categories (x-axis): Meat (g), Fruits (g), Vegetables (g), Potatoes (g), Breads & cereals (g), Eggs (g), Fat (%), Saturated fat (%), Alcohol (g), Fish (g), Legumes (g)

From: "Seven Countries: A multivariate analysis of death and coronary heart disease" A. Keys Harvard University Press 1980

straightforward way in which we can learn about the good or bad effects of the food we eat: Watch what people eat, and then see what they die from.

This kind of research lies at the very heart of the LifePoints system. It's not based on abstract theory. It's not trying to sell you the latest fad diet or trendy (but unproven) food supplement. It is, quite simply, utilizing the hard won results obtained from the longest running, most far-reaching experiment ever conducted in the history of the world. From North Pole to South, Far East to West, humans consume the most dramatically varied diets of any species on the face of the planet. Some of the foods we eat allow us to live out long lives with great vigor and vitality. Others seem to bestow little more than ill health and an early grave. We know enough now to begin to put this information to practical use.

And that's what LifePoints does.

LifePoints and RiskPoints— How They Work

The task of calculating LifePoints and RiskPoints numbers for each of the foods in this book began with a truly gigantic computational effort. Over the course of several months, computers performed countless millions of calculations day after day, night after night. Machines in both Europe and America, connected through the ubiquitous Internet, facilitated our effort.

Sometimes it seems that computers serve only to make our lives needlessly complicated. Yet without the awesome number-crunching power of today's computers this book could never have been possible. Gradually, the raw data began to take shape. For the first time, we began to see patterns emerging, and surprises too. Food that we had always believed to be "healthy" sometimes proved to be anything but. And frequently, we found ourselves bestowing new respect on modest foodstuffs that we'd hitherto disregarded. We're certain you will share these experiences as you become familiar with the LifePoints system. Indeed, we hope you share the thrill we first felt when you realize just how effective and uncomplicated it is to use. Sheer power over your diet—at your fingertips!

What do LifePoints actually measure? It's enough to remember that a food that has a high LifePoints number will provide you with a significant range of nutrients, in useful amounts. If that food is also low in RiskPoints, then it's safe to assume that it is a nutritionally valuable food that could, if you wish, form one of the core foods in your diet.

People sometimes expect the LifePoints system to be measured in calories or some other familiar unit, and are puzzled when it isn't. Well, think about it like this: Instead of measuring just one nutrient, LifePoints measures *lots* of them. First, we calculate an overall nutritional profile for the food being analyzed, in its most common serving size. Next, we use a proprietary computer algorithm to compare the nutritional profile of that food to its respective "ideal" nutritional profile, and see how it fits. A good fit earns lots of LifePoints, while a bad one earns none. It is important to emphasize that we're not just adding up all the nutrients in the food. That would produce a misleading result, since foods that contain very large amounts of just one or two nutrients would come out far too favorably. These two numbers—LifePoints and RiskPoints

—instantly provide you with a dynamic and enlightening picture of any food you care to look up! Now let's briefly describe the importance of the nutrients we've included in the LifePoints system.

What's the Good in LifePoints?

Beta-carotene

Is beta-carotene good for you, or a cause of cancer? Recently, there's been a lot of publicity about this particular nutrient, and it's left a great many people wondering whether they should be taking it or not. Actually, the beta-carotene dilemma is a perfect demonstration of the natural superiority of the LifePoints system. Because even though the uncertainty over beta-carotene won't finally be resolved for a decade or longer, LifePoints can help you make the correct decision *right now*—whatever the final verdict may be.

Let's start by defining what beta-carotene is. Simply, it's the plant form of vitamin A. Vitamin A (or retinol) was the first fat-soluble vitamin to be discovered, and is only found in certain animal tissues. Many Americans don't fully appreciate that retinol—which is often found in vitamin pills—can be toxic and teratogenic (in other words, it can cause fetal malformations if high doses are taken before or during pregnancy). Retinol's toxic effects can also include bone abnormalities and life-threatening liver damage. Dr. John Hathcock of the Food and Drug Administration estimates that 3 to 4 percent of the U.S. population take vitamin supplements containing large doses of retinol per day. "That's a heck of a lot of people," he comments. "If even 0.1 percent of the population are taking potentially toxic doses, that's too high."[9]

Fortunately, the plant kingdom is abundant in substances that are converted into vitamin A in the wall of the small intestine during digestion. These substances are sometimes called provitamin A, or carotenoids (sounds like "carrot," and indeed, carrots are a lavish source of carotenoids). Of the several hundred naturally occurring carotenoids, the most widespread and most active form is beta-carotene. And *unlike* retinol, foods that contain beta-carotene can be consumed in plentiful amounts *without* fear of toxicity. Also, beta-carotene is not teratogenic.[10] It is:

- Essential for good eyesight
- Vital for tissue growth and bone development
- Used to maintain the integrity of mucous membranes, thus building a barrier against infection
- Necessary for the proper growth and functioning of the reproductive system.

Over a hundred epidemiologic studies have shown that people who have high levels of beta-carotene in their diet, and in their blood, have considerably lower risks of cancer, particularly lung cancer.[11] That's why beta-carotene (but *not* retinol) is an important ingredient in the LifePoints number. In fact, it has been calculated that a diet richer in beta-carotene could save the lives of more than a third of the 400,000 Americans who die of cancer every year. In women, beta-carotene seems to be able to thwart cervical cancer. Further, epidemiological evidence indicates that it can also reduce the incidence of cancers of the larynx, bladder, esophagus, stomach, colorectum, and prostate gland.

Beta-carotene also functions as a powerful antioxidant and free radical quencher. Today, we hear a great deal about antioxidants and free radicals in the media. The LifePoints system delivers you a diet that is *naturally* high in many of the most powerful antioxidants. We'll explain why taking antioxidants in their *natural* form is important. First, let's describe what they are. In recent years, scientists have begun to appreciate just how crucial antioxidants are to our health.

In the popular media, free radicals are often characterized as "bad," but as in so many things, this is only partly true. The "free radical theory" was first proposed as long ago as 1954 by Dr. Denham Harman, former professor of medicine and biochemistry at the University of Nebraska. He discovered that radiation caused accelerated aging, and also created an excess of free radicals in body cells. What is a free radical? Simply, an atom or molecule with an unpaired electron. It is inherently unstable, as it continually searches for another molecule to which to attach itself. Gerontologist Alex Comfort wittily compared a free radical to a convention delegate away from his wife: "a highly reactive chemical agent that will combine with anything that's around." Free radicals trigger a chain reaction that "rusts" the body. They can damage cell membranes, proteins, carbohydrates, and deoxyribonucleic acid (DNA), the genetic material of the cell and of life itself. Up to now, some sixty diseases have been associated with free radical activity, including Alzheimer's, heart disease, arthritis, multiple sclerosis, and eye cataracts. Even "liver spots"—areas of brown skin that appear on your hands and arms later in life—are connected to the activity of free radicals. Although the body naturally produces free radicals, other substances, such as cigarette smoke, radiation, air pollution, herbicides, artificial flavorings, chlorine, rancid fats, alcohol, and toxic heavy metals, are also causes of free radical formation.

. . . .

TIP: Studies show that people who eat infrequently (one or two large meals daily) tend to put on more weight than people who eat more often. So don't feel guilty about snacking—it can be good for you. But do use the LifePoints system to make sure you're eating high-quality snacks.

. . . .

The process of aging isn't simply about crow's feet and turkey jowls—it actually brings about many serious changes in the human body. In fact, after the age of twenty-eight, the greatest single risk factor for disease and death is the aging process itself.[12] It is sobering to realize that, if one day all the major causes of premature death were eliminated, the average human lifespan would *still* be only eighty-five years.[13] The only way we're going to extend that is by modifying the aging process itself.

Human aging is by no means fully understood. But there's little doubt that one important aspect of the aging process is the damage that free radicals can inflict at the cellular level. It is when things get out of balance between free radicals (pro-oxidants) and antioxidants that problems begin. If you're low on antioxidants, then you're wide open to free radical attack. In fact, some scientists now suspect that what we call "aging" is simply the final result of many free radical reactions going on continuously through our cells and tissues.[14] If that view is correct, then aging might be amenable to alleviation, and what we today see as an inevitable process might, tomorrow, be considered to be a disease process—and treated accordingly.

Several scientific studies have already shown that dietary antioxidants can increase lifespan.[15] In America, the Alliance for Aging Research (a nonprofit public health organization) recently assembled a panel of leading medical researchers, nutritionists, and consumer safety experts to examine antioxidants and aging. They reviewed over 200 clinical and epidemiologic studies conducted over the past two decades and concluded that "A diet rich in antioxidants, including beta-carotene and vitamins C and E, is effective in guarding against heart disease, cancer, cataracts, and other conditions associated with aging."[16] LifePoints naturally provides you with a diet that is high in these major antioxidants.

However, free radicals aren't all bad. There is persuasive evidence that the basic chemicals of life first originated in the "primeval soup" from a series of free radical reactions, triggered by ionizing radiation from the sun. This would explain why free radical reactions are so pervasive in nature. They enable genetic mutations to occur, and thus play a pivotal role in the process of evolution. And your body *deliberately* produces free radicals when it wants to kill invading organisms, as part of its immune and inflammatory responses. Obviously, your body needs a way to *manage* free radicals effectively, and in particular, there has to be a protective and scavenging method to ensure that they don't get out of control. And that's what antioxidants such as beta-carotene can do superbly.

Of course, the key question is: If all these studies show that beta-carotene is so good for us, why is it also suspected of promoting cancer? This doubt was first raised when the results of a long-awaited major study came to the startling conclusion that high doses of synthetic beta-carotene, when taken in pill form, may sometimes *raise* the risk of cancer rather than lower it.[17] The ten-year, $43 million study was conducted on 29,133 male cigarette smokers who lived in Finland—smokers were chosen because they are already at high risk of lung cancer. The findings were disturbing in two ways: First, they indicated that beta-carotene supplements had little or no effect (good or bad) on the incidence of any cancer apart from lung cancer; but in the case of lung cancer, those people taking the pills seemed to *increase* their lung cancer risk by 18 percent.

Puzzling indeed, particularly since the only previous large-scale clinical trial had produced precisely the opposite results (taking a combination of beta-carotene, vitamin E, and selenium pills has been shown to reduce deaths from stomach cancer by 21 percent among 15,000 people living in Linxian County in China).[18] And now, even more confusingly, a twelve-year study, recently completed, seems to show that beta-carotene pills have *no* effect on the incidence of cancer or heart disease—good or bad.[19] So what on earth can we conclude from this seemingly contradictory information? No wonder people are bewildered!

Studies such as these typically take years, even decades, to produce results. In the meantime, what are we to think? Well, the LifePoints system can help guide you through even this dietary chaos. Let's assume the worst possible scenario, in other words, that the findings of the Finnish study are correct. What would they actually mean to us, in practice? The Finnish study examined the effect of giving *synthetic* beta-carotene in pill form to people who had been smokers for a long time. We could therefore conclude that long-term smokers shouldn't take synthetic beta-carotene vitamin pills (and most multivitamin pills do contain synthetic beta-carotene). However, we should *not* conclude that naturally rich food sources of beta-carotene should be avoided. As we've just mentioned, more than a hundred separate studies now show that people who consume foods naturally rich in beta-carotene have considerably lower risks of cancer. One typical investigation followed the health of 1,556 middle-aged men employed by the Western Electric Company, and found that those who consumed the greatest amounts of beta-carotene-rich foods slashed their risk of dying of cancer by 40 percent, and their risk of dying from heart disease by 30 percent.[20] Decades of studies tracking the health of thousands of people prove the wisdom of eating beta-carotene-rich foods. But whether it's wise to replace this sort of food with a synthetic pill—well that's very much open to question.

And there are certainly plenty of questions right now. Why should foods rich in beta-carotene reduce the risk of lung cancer, while high doses of beta-carotene supplements seem to increase it? Perhaps massive doses of synthetic beta-carotene prevent us from absorbing other substances in foods that may be the real cancer protectors? Perhaps beta-carotene can only work as a cancer defense when functioning in combination with its naturally occurring carotenoid brethren, such as alpha-carotene, lutein, zeaxanthin, cryptoxanthin, lycopene, and hundreds of other carotenoids?

These questions, and many more, will take time to answer. But the beauty of the LifePoints system is this: You don't have to wait for the final, conclusive answers before using the system for your immediate benefit. You see, we already know that foods that rate high for beta-carotene are also strongly associated with many substantial health benefits, such as reduced cancer and heart disease risks. Whether these health benefits are *due to* the beta-carotene content of the food, or whether beta-carotene is simply a *marker* for a far more complex and as yet undiscovered nutritional health factor is immaterial to the functioning of the LifePoints system—it doesn't really matter. Look at it like this: You don't need to have a degree in aerodynamics in order to buy a plane ticket. All you need to know is that the plane flies and will get you to your destination.

Remember: No nutrient works in isolation in nature. The natural beta-carotene content of a food is one—but only one—component of the LifePoints number. The LifePoints system gives you a unique way of assessing the broad nutritional profile of many different kinds of foods, and lets you compare one food with another.

Vitamin C

While vitamin C was long considered relevant only to the prevention of scurvy, there is now abundant evidence that a diet rich in vitamin C can help to prevent a wide range of human diseases. Humans are one of the few species unable to synthesize vitamin C internally, and therefore we need to be certain of a regular, high-quality dietary intake. Vitamin C is also a very effective antioxidant and free radical quencher. You can even see it at work for yourself in a simple experiment. Cut an apple in half, and put one half aside. Pour lemon juice, which is high in vitamin C, on the other half. The half without the lemon juice will go brown through oxidation much faster than the half protected by the antioxidant vitamin C. In a recent study conducted at the University of California at Berkeley, scientists isolated plasma from human blood, incubated it at body temperature, and added a chemical that is known to produce free radicals as it decomposes. When vitamin C was added, it neutralized 100 percent of the free radicals generated.[21] Vitamin C also:

- Assists in the production of collagen, a protein that is the body's building block for all connective tissue, cartilage, bones, teeth, skin, and tendons
- Helps wounds, fractures, bruises, and hemorrhages heal
- Maintains function of immune system
- Greatly facilitates the absorption of iron from the diet
- Assists hemoglobin and red blood cell production
- Is an essential cofactor for metabolism of many other nutrients
- Helps the body cope with physiological and psychological stress.

Further, Vitamin C seems to block the formation of nitrosamines. Nitrates and nitrites are added to foods to give color and flavor, and to act as preservatives. During digestion these substances are converted by the human body into nitrosamines, which are known to be powerful cancer-causing chemicals (they are particularly associated with cancers of the stomach and esophagus). The good news is that if a vitamin-C-rich food is taken at the same time as foods containing nitrates or nitrites, the production of nitrosamines is greatly reduced. But perhaps you could achieve the same sort of dietary benefit simply by taking a vitamin C supplement? Well, no. As in the case of beta-carotene, the beauty of the LifePoints system is that it doesn't *just* measure the amount of vitamin C in your diet. LifePoints uses the vitamin C content of food as a *marker* for other health-enhancing nutrients, yet to be identified, in a foodstuff. We can explain this by referring to a rather elegantly designed experiment recently conducted at Cornell University.[22] Scientists examined nitrosamine formation in human subjects by giving one group of people fruit juices to drink, and another group the same amount of purified vitamin C in supplement form. The study ran for sixteen days, during which time the subjects' urine was analyzed for nitrosamine activity. The results clearly showed that the group taking the fruit juices was producing fewer nitrosamines than the group consuming the same amount of purified vitamin C in supplement form. Green pepper, tomato, pineapple, strawberry, and carrot juice were found to be particularly effective at inhibiting nitrosamine formation. Clearly, vitamin C is an important antinitrosamine dietary factor, but it is *most* effective when working in combination with even more powerful—and as yet unidentified—natural dietary substances. Because the LifePoints number uses vitamin C as one of its markers for a food's nutritional profile, we can take advantage of research such as this today, even though the precise biochemical mechanism may remain unidentified for many years to come.

It has also been found that women with abnormal cervical smear results often have low amounts of vitamin C in their bodies.[23] This may shed new light on the underlying damage caused by smoking, because it has long been established that women who smoke have higher levels of cervical cancer. Smoking impairs the absorption of vitamin C but smoking also requires that you take more vitamin C to minimize its effects as a pollutant.

Thiamin

Also called thiamine or vitamin B_1, thiamin was discovered to be the nutritional factor responsible for preventing the disease *beriberi* (Singhalese for "I cannot," meaning that the sufferer is too ill to do anything). Epidemics of beriberi occurred in Asia as a result of eating a diet of white polished rice, in which all the nutritional content of the outer layers of rice is discarded during processing. Although beriberi is primarily a disease of tropical countries, nutritional deficiencies of thiamin are also seen in the West, especially among people who typically eat a highly refined junk food diet. In the body, thiamin functions to:

- Convert carbohydrate into energy for muscles and nervous system
- Keep mucous membranes healthy

- Maintain a positive mental state and possibly assist in learning capacity.

Riboflavin

Also known as vitamin B_2, riboflavin was first observed in 1879 as a greenish fluorescent pigment present in milk, but its function was not fully understood until 1932. It is often found in combination with other B-group vitamins, and since it is not stored in the human body for any period of time, it is vital that your diet supply regular amounts. A deficiency will result in cracked and scaly skin; soreness of lips, mouth, and tongue; and sometimes heightened sensitivity to light, watering of eyes, or conjunctivitis. In the body, riboflavin works:

- With other vitamins and enzymes in the utilization of energy from food
- To keep mucous membranes healthy
- As a key component in normal tissue respiration.

Niacin

Also called vitamin B_3, niacin is the collective name for nicotinamide (niacinamide) and nicotinic acid. Its importance was recognized in 1937 when it was discovered that the disease pellagra was caused by niacin deficiency. Lack of niacin in the diet can also lead to fatigue and muscle weakness, loss of appetite, and mental unbalance. In the body, it plays an important role in:

- The release of energy from carbohydrates, fats, and proteins
- DNA synthesis
- Keeping the skin, nerves, and digestive system working healthily.

Vitamin B_6

Also known as pyridoxine, vitamin B_6 is (in common with other B-group vitamins) soluble in water. This means that the body's storage capacity for B_6 is limited, and we need to ensure a good daily dietary intake. It works in the body to:

- Manufacture and convert amino acids and metabolize protein
- Produce hemoglobin
- Convert the amino acid tryptophan to niacin
- Facilitate the release of glycogen for energy from the liver and muscles
- Help the body process linoleic acid (an essential fatty acid)
- Help build and maintain the integrity of the nervous system and brain.

Vitamin B_{12}

Also called cobalamin, this vitamin is manufactured by microorganisms such as yeasts, bacteria, molds, and some algae. The human body can store this vitamin for considerable periods (five or six years) so a daily dietary source is not essential. In addition, the healthy body recycles this vitamin very effectively, recovering it from bile and other intestinal secretions, which is why the dietary requirement is so low (being measured in millionths of a gram). However, B_{12} deficiency is an occasional problem for people on restricted diets, and in view of its importance, it is wise to consume a known B_{12} food source from time to time. Its functions in the body are to:

- Facilitate the normal metabolic function of all cells
- Work with folate to prevent anemia
- Assist in the process of DNA synthesis
- Promote the growth and normal functioning of the nervous system.

Folate

Folate and folacin (sometimes called vitamin B_9) are the names used to describe a group of substances chemically similar to folic acid. Its importance to growth and the prevention of anemia was established in 1946. The word *folate* comes from the Latin word *folium,* meaning a leaf, which should tell us something about the best sources of this vitamin. In the body, it:

- Plays an essential role in the formation of DNA and RNA

- Functions together with vitamin B_{12} in amino acid synthesis
- Is essential for the formation of red and white blood cells
- Contributes to the formation of the iron constituent of hemoglobin.

Calcium

The most plentiful mineral in the human body, calcium amounts to three and a half pounds or so of the average adult's weight. Ninety-nine percent is deposited in the bones and teeth, with the remainder fulfilling essential regulatory functions in the blood and cellular fluids. The body stores its skeletal calcium in two ways: in the nonexchangeable pool (calcium, which is on "long-term deposit" in the bones) and in the exchangeable pool, which can act as a short-term buffer to smooth over the peaks and troughs in day-to-day dietary calcium intakes. If dietary intake is consistently too low, then the exchangeable pool of calcium will become so depleted that the calcium on "long-term deposit" in the bones will be put to use, thus inducing bone degeneration.

Although calcium is often thought of as the "bone mineral," the 1 percent of serum calcium in the human body (calcium held outside the skeletal structure) is responsible for a vital and complex range of tasks. Calcium is clearly a critical nutrient, and we all need to ensure that we get it. Many people erroneously believe that the consumption of heroic quantities of dairy products is the only way to prevent bone-depleting afflictions such as osteoporosis. This is not so. A major study of the Chinese population reveals that they take in only half the amount of calcium that Westerners do, but osteoporosis is very rare in China.[24] Why should this be? Well, most Chinese eat no dairy products and instead get all their calcium from vegetables. This is why we've included the calcium content of all foods as another marker in the LifePoints number. We'd like you to get a good calcium intake from a wide variety of foods, rather than assuming that large amounts of milk and dairy products will protect you. Calcium also functions in the body to:

- Help build and maintain bones and teeth
- Help control transport of chemicals across cell membranes
- Facilitate the release of neurotransmitters at synapses
- Influence the function of protein hormones and enzymes
- Help regulate heartbeat and muscle tone
- Initiate blood clotting.

Iron

We all know that iron prevents anemia, and is essential for hemoglobin production. As such, it is involved in the transport of oxygen from the lungs to the body's tissues, it transports and stores oxygen in the muscles, and is involved in the proper functioning of the immune system and intellect. Iron deficiency is the most common of all deficiency diseases in both developing and developed countries. Scientists vary in their estimate of what precisely constitutes a state of iron depletion, but the general cutoff point is variously calculated to lie between 12 and 25 micrograms of ferritin (one of the chief iron storage forms) per liter of plasma.

. . . .

TIP: Study after study indicates that the slower you lose weight, the more likely you are to actually lose fat rather than muscle tissue. Also, weight lost slowly is more likely to be kept off permanently.

. . . .

Iron is well conserved by the body (90 percent of the 3 to 5 grams in our bodies is continually recycled). The major cause of iron depletion is loss of blood itself—as in menstruation, which on average causes about half a milligram of iron to be lost for every day of the period. However, this can vary very widely (losses as high as 1.4 mg a day have been reported) so the official recommended daily allowances for women attempt to take this into account by building in a generous safety margin. For example, an iron intake of 10.8 mg a day appears to meet the needs of 86 percent of all menstruating women,[25] yet the official American recommended daily allowance has been set at 15 mg a day in an attempt to meet the needs of the remaining 14 percent. This is, in fact, an uneasy compromise, because even at this level of iron consumption, 5 percent of women who have very heavy periods will not have an adequate intake to replace losses. The rate of absorption of iron from the diet can be significantly affected, for better or worse, by several factors:

- The rate of iron absorption is controlled by the degree to which iron is actually *needed* by the body. Normally, only 5 to 15 percent of the iron in food is actually absorbed, but this can rise to 50 percent in cases of iron deficiency.
- Foods containing vitamin C will considerably increase iron absorption. Iron must be delivered in a soluble form to the small intestine if it is to be absorbed, and vitamin C can make sure that the iron found in plant foods remains soluble in the acidic environment normally found there. Other organic acids found in fruit and vegetables, such as malic acid and citric acid, are also thought to possess this iron-enhancing attribute. This effect is substantial: Adding 60 mg of vitamin C to a meal of rice has been shown to more than triple the absorption of iron; adding the same amount to a meal of corn enhances absorption fivefold. The LifePoints number includes both iron and vitamin C as markers.
- The tannin in tea can significantly reduce the absorption of iron by combining with it to form insoluble iron compounds. The food preservative EDTA can also exercise the same inhibitory effect. Both of these factors can reduce assimilation by as much as 50 percent.

Zinc

The human body contains a mere 2 grams of zinc, distributed in the tissues in varying concentrations. Its importance to good human nutrition has only been recognized in recent times (the first reports appeared in 1963). Low zinc status often manifests itself in a decrease in the senses of taste and smell, delays in healing, and failure to grow properly. This is because, in the human body, zinc is:

- An essential component of many enzymes that work with red blood cells to transport carbon dioxide from tissues to lungs
- A vital factor in many key life processes, such as our immune function and the expression of genetic information.

In addition to all the key nutrients mentioned above, the LifePoints number also assesses foods for their fiber content (which as you must know, imparts a whole host of health benefits, ranging from the prevention of various forms of cancer to lowering blood cholesterol and preventing constipation) and their protein content. *A high LifePoints number indicates that the food concerned is a plentiful source of the nutrients mentioned above. A low number indicates that it is a poor source.*

When you consider that the LifePoints system rates foods for all the above nutrients, and ensures that you don't consume dangerous levels of the unhealthy ingredients, you can see why we say that LifePoints is "beyond calories." Just imagine: What would happen if all the world were to eat a natural diet high in LifePoints and low in RiskPoints? Actually, we don't have to imagine. The science of epidemiology already suggests what many of the benefits could be. Here they are:

- Bolstering the immune system
- Preventing coronary heart disease
- Reversing coronary heart disease
- Preventing cancers
- Delaying the aging process
- Preventing cataracts
- Preventing osteoporosis
- Preventing and treating high blood pressure
- Preventing strokes
- Preventing impotence
- Preventing and treating obesity
- Treating arthritis
- Preventing gout
- Preventing and treating diabetes
- Preventing hypoglycemia
- Preventing and treating constipation
- Preventing varicose veins
- Preventing appendicitis
- Preventing gallstones
- Reducing food poisoning

Sounds like a pretty healthy world, doesn't it?

What's the Bad in RiskPoints?

There is one unequivocal risk factor in the diets most of us eat today, and that is the amount of fat consumed. Fat—and in particular saturated fat (mainly from animal sources)—is without doubt our number one dietary enemy today. Most of us already know that eating too much fatty food is supposed to be bad for us. But we'll bet you *didn't* know these shocking and startling facts:

- **Eating 100 calories from fat will make you put on more weight than eating 100 calories from carbohydrates.** On the face of it, this seems impossible. After all, 100 calories is 100 calories, no matter where it comes from—right? Wrong! Your body stores surplus energy intake in the form of fat. When you eat fatty foods, your body can very easily and very efficiently turn that food fat into body fat. Only about 3 percent of the fat you consume is burned up by your body in the storage process.[26] Building massive hips and thighs has never been easier! However, the process of turning carbohydrate-rich foods into body fat consumes a considerable proportion (about 25 percent) of their calories. Further, carbohydrate-rich meals will boost your body's metabolism, which in turn makes it harder for you to gain weight. Fatty foods simply don't have this effect.

- **If you want to control your weight, all types of fat are equally bad.** Forget the advertising slogans about polyunsaturates and monounsaturates. None of them help you shed those pounds. One gram of fat—of any kind—yields twice as many calories as a gram of protein or a gram of carbohydrate. Fat is a poor nutritional return on your food investment.

- **A naturally low-fat diet can do remarkable things, including reverse heart disease.** Scientifically, there's no remaining doubt. The plaque that builds up and eventually blocks coronary arteries can be unblocked by eating a good, low-fat diet. Among other benefits, increased flow of blood in these arteries can also reduce the pain of angina.[27]

One simple RiskPoints number manages to achieve two important goals with regard to fat. First, it ensures that your *total* fat consumption remains healthily low. How low? Well, if your RiskPoints daily total adds up to no more than 100, you'll have eaten no more than 40 grams of fat. This is the sort of intake that research shows our species has *naturally consumed* for most of our history. In many parts of the world—China, for example—people still consume this (to us) relatively low level of fat in their diets. The result? Many of the "diseases of civilization" that so plague us in the West are virtually unknown there. Why do we suggest you keep your fat intake down to this level? Here's how the *New York Times* put it when reporting the results of the largest ever scientific study into the diets and health of the Chinese people: "Reducing dietary fat to less than 30 percent of calories, as is currently recommended for Americans, *may not be enough* to curb the risk of heart disease and cancer. To make a significant impact, the Chinese data imply, a maximum of 20 percent of calories from fat—and preferably only 10 to 15 percent—should be consumed."[28] The "China Study" is a turning point in the science of epidemiology. The study began in 1983, with the aim of exploring the dietary causes of cancer. Since then, it has been expanded to include heart, metabolic, and infectious diseases. And these findings are only the beginning. Professor T. Colin Campbell, a nutritional biochemist from Cornell University and the American mastermind of the study, predicts that this "living laboratory" will continue to generate vital findings for the next forty to fifty years. Already, the China Study has confirmed that obesity is clearly related to *what* you eat, rather than how much. The Chinese actually consume 20 percent *more* calories than Westerners do, but Westerners are 25 percent fatter! The culprit? All that fat in our food.

Keep your RiskPoints to round about 100, and you'll be eating a naturally low-fat diet. But that's by no means all it does for you. The RiskPoints number also intelligently guides you *away* from food unhealthily high in saturated fat, and steers you *toward* food low in it. Why is this important? Because saturated fat is clearly linked to the development of coronary heart disease, and probably to certain cancers, too. In this respect, all fat is *not* the same. We don't want you getting all your fat intake as unhealthy saturated fat. So the RiskPoints formula penalizes foods that are too high in this type of fat. You can think of this part of the RiskPoints equation as a silent friend there in the background, gently nudging you away from unhealthy foods and leading you to the healthier choices. You may not notice it, but it's there, working for you all the time!

Putting LifePoints To Work

If you can count to one hundred, you can use Life-Points! Let's show you how. Then we'll answer some of the common questions people often have.

All the foods listed in this book have been carefully and painstakingly analyzed to reveal their overall nutritional profile. Each food has two numbers:

- **The LifePoints number is a measure of the food's healthy components—the higher the number, the healthier the food.**
- **The RiskPoints number is a measure of the food's unhealthy components—the higher the number, the more unhealthy the food.**

So a food with high RiskPoints and no LifePoints is a "bad" food. Similarly, a food with high LifePoints and no RiskPoints is a "good" food. Your aim is to maximize the number of LifePoints you consume and minimize the RiskPoints. How many Risk-Points and LifePoints should you consume? It's simple:

Your LifePoints should total at least 100 per day
Your RiskPoints should total no more than 100 per day

That's all the adding up you have to do! Now you know the way the LifePoints system works. It's much easier than calorie counting, because you don't have to add up to 1000 or more. And, uniquely, the Life-Points system gives you a feeling for the food itself. Use it for just a day or two, and you'll find that your own instincts for good food and bad food are revived and developed. That's why we say LifePoints is an empowering system.

Now we'd like to give you some guidelines that will enable you to use the system most effectively:

1. For your convenience, the foods are divided into six major groups, and there's a comprehensive index at the back as well. To eat a healthy and varied diet, you must choose foods from the first four groups. Groups 5 and 6 are optional. The suggested number of servings per day from each group is listed below:

Group 1	Fruit and Fruit Juices	3 servings
Group 2	Cereals, Grains, and Pasta	4 servings
Group 3	Vegetables and Vegetable Products	4 servings
Group 4	Legumes, Nuts, and Seeds	3 servings
Group 5	Meat, Fish, and Dairy	optional
Group 6	Drinks, Desserts, Snacks, and Sauces	optional

2. Variety is the keynote of healthy eating. So to encourage you to eat as wide a variety as possible, please observe the following rule:

The LifePoints for any foodstuff can only be counted once, no matter how often you eat that food during the day. This means that if you eat the same food twice, only its RiskPoints count for the second helping. In other words, don't try to cheat the system by eating ten servings of broccoli for 120 LifePoints and only 10 RiskPoints! (Using this simple rule, if you ever did eat ten helpings of broccoli, you'd accumulate 10 RiskPoints but only 12 LifePoints.)

3. Foods are listed in common serving sizes, but it's quite acceptable to halve or even quarter the servings, providing that you also reduce the associated RiskPoints and LifePoints.

People are not always used to sitting down and planning their day's diet—too often our food consumption is the last thing we think about, when it really should be the first—and sometimes it's not easy to decide where to begin. Well, now it is easy!

Answers to All Your Questions

We've found that when people start using the Life-Points system, the same sorts of questions often crop up. Here they are, together with the answers.

- -

TIP: There's no need to weigh yourself every day. Everyone experiences small fluctuations in weight, and small increases discourage you, deterring healthy eating habits. Pay more attention to how fit you feel, rather than what the scales say.

- -

Do I have to make allowances for the freshness of food?

Food quality is a very important issue to us. The level of nutrition you receive from your diet depends not only on what food you choose to eat, but also, among other things, on how you store and cook it. This provides at least three opportunities for nutrient loss. If you lead a hectic, demanding life, you need these nutrients even more, and therefore need to know how you can safeguard them. Please read and note the advice that follows:

Choice of food

The more a foodstuff is processed, the greater the loss of natural nutrients. So buy only unprocessed foods.

If possible, buy organic foods, preferably from local

producers. These are more likely to have their nutrients intact and, if they are from local sources, they will not have been in long storage during transit. Nutrients decay with time, so eat close to the soil!

Also, the risk of pesticide residue is remote. Pesticides are poisons—their basic purpose is to kill. In an ideal world, there should be no pesticide residue on food by the time it reaches consumers, but considerable evidence indicates that the food we eat *can* be tainted with pesticide residue, even if it's been washed many times.

Farmers spend twice as much on herbicides as they do on insecticides and fungicides put together. Many of these herbicides are designed to be absorbed directly into the plant's system, so it is impossible to get rid of them simply by washing.

Another worrying fact: Ten years ago, scientists exposed a statistical connection between the use of herbicides and Parkinson's disease, which affects the central nervous system in humans.[29]

So what is organic food? Well, it's food that is produced responsibly, taking account of the needs of consumers, farm animals, and the environment. Organic farmers produce food that:

- Is grown without artificial pesticides and fertilizers
- Tastes good rather than just looks good
- Is never irradiated
- Contains no artificial hormones, genetically manipulated organisms, or unnecessary medication
- Is not overprocessed

- Does not contain flavorings, dyes, and other additives
- Is nutritious and promotes positive health and well-being.

Organic food is also better for the environment. Intensive agriculture is responsible for about 50 percent of all water pollution (such as high nitrate levels). It has been clearly established that modern biological-organic farming methods result in less leaching of nitrates into the water supply and lower nitrate content in vegetables.

Here are some guidelines for purchasing foods:

- Do check the "use-by" date. Old produce will have suffered severe nutritional decay. Shopkeepers always put older stock at the front of the display, so buy from the back.
- Canning and bottling reduces the levels of vitamin C, thiamin, and folic acid. Vitamin C loss continues during storage. If you have to buy canned food, do not keep it overlong. Although it may be safe to eat, its nutrients may be severely depleted.
- Avoid foods that contain sulfur dioxide as a preservative—they will have almost entirely lost their thiamin (vitamin B_1) content.
- Freeze-dried foods are relatively good since their nutrients have not been depleted by heating.
- Frozen foods suffer some thiamin and vitamin C loss. However, the loss is less than in fresh food that has been kept for a number of days. If shopping for

fresh food is a problem for you, frozen foods are probably the next best alternative, but be very careful not to overcook them (see below).

- Choose unrefined monounsaturated oils—preferably olive oil—for cooking. Pure, refined polyunsaturated oils turn rancid more easily.

Don't buy foods in damaged cans, no matter how good a bargain they appear to be. Small cracks in the can lining will affect the delicate vitamins and other nutrients and may even cause the food itself to turn bad.

Storage

- Store oils, fats, and oily foods like cheeses and shelled nuts in the refrigerator. This will help to slow down the process of oxidation, which turns them rancid.

- Vitamin C, thiamin, riboflavin, and folic acid all decay quickly in air. Once vegetables are harvested, the damaged tissues release an enzyme that starts to destroy the vitamin C. Blanching inhibits the enzyme, which is why freezing fresh vegetables is much better than keeping them unfrozen and eating them many days later.

- Vegetables lose around 70 percent of their folic acid content within 3 days if they are stored in daylight. Store vegetables in the refrigerator until you are ready to use them, or freeze them immediately.

- Store grains and cereals whole in a dry, cool place.

Cooking

- Cooking is generally harmful to the nutrients in food. However, it also changes starches, proteins, and some vitamins into accessible forms for us as well as releasing nutrients otherwise bound into certain foods, like the amino acid tryptophan in cornmeal. Cooking is necessary to destroy toxic substances in such foods as soybeans and kidney beans. Cooking also makes some foods, like meat, palatable to eat. However, there are ways in which you can reduce the nutrient loss in foods during the cooking process.

- Pressure-cooking is perhaps the best way to reduce nutrient loss. Invest in a nonaluminum pressure cooker which, because of the reduced cooking times, will also reduce energy consumption and therefore the size of your fuel bills.

- After pressure-cooking, steaming and microwave cooking are the next healthiest options. (A steamer is obviously a lot cheaper than a microwave oven!) Further down the list are, in order of preference:
  - Boiling
  - Grilling
  - Stir frying (at high temperature where the fat seals in the nutrients)
  - Sautéing
  - Deep-frying

- If you cook with fat, don't let it become so hot that it starts to smoke. At this temperature the essential fatty acid linoleic acid is destroyed immediately.

- Fats that have been used for cooking once must be discarded, since the linoleic acid and vitamins A and C will have been lost.
- If you boil food, do so for the minimum amount of time and then use the water for stock afterward. The fragile water-soluble vitamins as well as some minerals leach into cooking water, which is why soups are so nutritious.
- Don't add baking soda to cooking water, even if you see it recommended for cooking certain types of legumes. It destroys valuable B vitamins.
- Prepare food immediately before cooking—remember that vitamin C is destroyed once vegetable cells are damaged. For the same reason, try not to chop them too finely. Scrubbing vegetables is better than peeling them.
- Once they are prepared, immerse the vegetables in boiling water immediately.
- Use pans with close-fitting lids and avoid using copper pans, which encourage oxidation and vitamin C loss.
- Once food is cooked, eat it at once. Keeping it warm will only result in further nutrient loss. That is why eating out too frequently may be less than healthy for you.

If you lead a hectic life and believe you don't have time for some of the advice given above, think again. The life you lead is totally dependent on a good nutritional support system, without which you're just running on empty. And you can only do that for so long.

Shopping regularly for fresh foods can appear to present a problem if you don't attach a very high priority to it. But just think: no sensible person buys a Rolls-Royce and then tries to run it on the cheapest gasoline! It's the same with your body—the better the fuel, the better the performance.

Do I have to follow the measurements given?

The more accurate you can be with your measurements, the better the system will work for you. To make things as easy as possible, most of the foods are listed in common measurements (a cup, a slice, and so on). Remember, we want you to eat as widely as possible. Do you know what the prime cause of malnutrition is? Most people in the West often erroneously believe that it's lack of food, but that's not true. The principal cause of malnutrition is lack of *variety* of food. A monotonous diet is a dangerous diet. To encourage you to choose as widely as possible, we suggest:

- If you want to eat *less* than the stated serving size, simply divide the LifePoints and RiskPoints appropriately (e.g. if you eat half the serving size, simply divide them by 2).
- If you want to eat *more* than the stated serving size, multiply the RiskPoints appropriately (e.g. if you eat twice the serving size, multiply the RiskPoints by 2) but the LifePoints *stay unchanged*.

How accurate are the numbers?

We've used food values collected from the world's leading authorities for our calculations. The major variable is, inevitably, the quality and freshness of the food concerned (see above). However, let's also realize that men and women don't live by numbers alone. At the end of the day, the most important function the LifePoints and RiskPoints figures serve is to awaken in you your own instinctive sense for what a healthy diet is. And that's the best possible use for the LifePoints system. We don't want you to be a slave to the numbers, we want you to use them to educate and liberate!

Can't I just subtract the RiskPoints from the LifePoints to produce one simple number?

In a word, no. When we were first developing the system, we tried very hard to achieve this. But because they are essentially two completely different measures of a food's worth, it is not possible to combine them meaningfully. Besides, we think having two numbers is actually superior to having one. This is why: Either number alone tells you very little about the good and bad ingredients in a foodstuff. What enables you to get a feel for the food concerned is to see the ratio of positive and negative elements in it. When you've used the system for a day or two, you'll see what we mean.

What happens if I exceed my daily RiskPoints?

Don't worry, you won't drop dead! However, it's a strong indication that you're not eating the healthiest diet you could. Just try to gradually get those Risk-Points down to 100 or so. It may take some time to reeducate your taste buds, particularly if you're used to a high-fat diet, but that's what life's all about! Don't feel dejected if you can't hit the 100 mark instantly. The LifePoints system is a tool; use it as you would any other to achieve your success over a period of time. "Success by the inch is a cinch—by the yard, it's hard!"

If I hit 100 daily LifePoints, does it guarantee that I've got all my recommended daily allowances?

Recommended daily allowances (RDAs), like calories, can be misleading. One of the most dangerous things they do is give people a false sense of security that they're well nourished. RDAs are, in reality, "best guesses" by a panel of government officials. When the U.S. Department of Agriculture released its "dietary pyramid," the eminent nutritional authority Walter C. Willett, of the Harvard School of Public Health, had this to say about it in *Science* magazine:

> Inevitably, such a document represents a mix of well-supported findings, educated guesses, and

political compromises with powerful economic interests such as the dairy and meat industries.[30]

Another problem with RDAs is that they're entirely impossible for ordinary people to use. Just adding up your daily food intake for *one* nutrient is difficult enough, but when you have to cope with a dozen or more, and watch your fat, and calories, and endlessly juggle your daily menus to make sure you hit all your RDAs—forget it! Ultimately, trying to follow any RDA system leads to one thing only (apart, that is, from madness!): pills. That's the only way you can *guarantee* that you're getting 100 percent of the recommended daily intake of specific vitamins and minerals. And as we've already seen (under beta-carotene), pills are *not* a substitute for a healthy diet.

....

TIP: Don't worry if your rate of weight loss slows down or stops from time to time. If you hit a plateau like this, don't cut back on your food intake—your body will think you're in a starvation situation. Stick to the same food consumption, but perhaps gently increase your exercise schedule, and you'll find weight loss will resume.

....

We don't want you to hit 100 LifePoints and then sit back. See if you can get it higher—write to us, and tell us how high. The RDA approach implies that a certain (guestimated) level of nutrition is all you need to bother with. Increasingly, this assumption is being challenged and discredited as old science. The LifePoints system goes far beyond RDAs. By showing you the good, high-nutrient foods and steering you away from the empty or hazardous foods, it gives you the big picture. Eating a high-quality diet is far more important than worrying whether your vitamin C consumption is 55 grams or 60 grams. And that's what LifePoints can do for you.

I eat out a lot, how can I cope in restaurants?

The same way you'd cope at home or in the supermarket. Use LifePoints to help you choose good food. Beware sauces, dressings, and other easily overlooked, "invisible" foods. You'll find them all listed in the LifePoints chart, so there's no excuse to go to pieces.

I've heard that plants contain natural chemicals that cause cancer, so nothing's really safe to eat, is it?

Yes, some plants certainly do produce chemicals to defend themselves against fungi, insects, and animal predators. Consider the cabbage. It contains forty-nine natural pesticides and metabolites, many of which may be cancer-causing or cancer-promoting. Actually, it's been estimated that there are between five thousand and ten thousand natural pesticides and associated breakdown products in our diets. And we eat about 1.5 grams of them every day. But wait. Before you decide to give up eating for good, consider this. Even though people who eat cabbages are certainly taking in all those natural pesticides that the cabbage uses to defend itself, those same people actually have a *greatly reduced* risk of getting cancer. Further, research shows that cabbage may actually retard existing cancers from spreading (metastasis). So what's going on? Simply this. *Nothing works in isolation.* A naturally healthy diet contains more than enough life-protecting nutrients and other factors to block the effect of minor plant toxins. So don't give up on the cabbage.

Where does alcohol fit in to the system?

Our advice is to restrict your alcohol consumption to the occasional glass of red wine. In most countries, high dietary intakes of saturated fats are strongly associated with high coronary heart disease death rates. Some regions of France, however, are an important exception to this rule; they have low heart disease death rates despite high-fat diets. This paradox is probably due to the antioxidant phenolic compounds that red wine contains (and as we all know, the French *do* drink red wine). No other alcohol has this effect.

Why are meat, fish, and dairy products an optional group?

Simply because considerable research shows that people who don't eat these products are healthier than those who do. One major scientific study followed the health of 25,000 Americans for twenty years, and found that meat consumption correlated very precisely with the risk of developing fatal heart disease.[31] People consuming meat only one or two days a week are 44 percent more likely to die from heart disease compared to those who don't eat meat, and people eating it between three and five times a week are 60 percent more likely to die. For men in one particular age group—forty-five to fifty-four—the risk seems to be particularly high. For these people—prime candidates for heart disease—the risk, when they are compared to nonmeat eaters, is 400 percent greater. Another study, this one from Japan, confirms these findings: In this case, the diets and health of 122,261 people were tracked over sixteen years.[32] Two life-styles emerged as being very high risk and very low risk respectively. The key risk factors in the high-risk life-style were smoking, drinking, meat consumption, and not eating green vegetables. The low-risk life-style was, not surprisingly, precisely the opposite. Interestingly, simply adding one factor—meat consumption—to an otherwise healthy life-style had a serious effect on mortality. The difference between the lowest risk group (no smoking, no drinking, no meat, and lots of green vegetables) and those people who led a similar life-style *except for eating meat* was that the meat-eaters boosted their risk of dying from heart disease by 30 percent—just by adding meat to an otherwise healthy lifestyle!

As far as cancer is concerned, the picture is much

the same. A major British twelve-year tracking study from the London School of Hygiene and Tropical Medicine has found that meat consumption increases the risk of dying from any form of cancer by a serious 40 percent, and a great many other studies have come to the same conclusions.[33] Of course, this is a highly political issue, as the American Cancer Society found when it recently announced revised dietary guidelines that called for a curtailment of red meat consumption, to the ire of the meat industry.[34] Study after study shows that we need to refocus our diets to become higher in fruits, vegetables, and whole grains, and lower in high-fat foods, especially those containing animal fats. LifePoints can help you to achieve this easily. But as with all things, LifePoints is your *tool*— it guides, but it doesn't compel.

I'm not just fat, I'm flabby. What can I do about that?

Skin is elastic and after a time it will tighten up. But you can help it and your muscles by doing regular exercise. Join a local fitness or yoga class to use all of your muscles in a gentle, gradual stretching regimen. Your muscles will alter shape as a result and you will regain some of the curves and corners you used to be so proud of. Alternatively, take up walking as your form of fitness training. Brisk, determined walking is actually an aerobic exercise that helps you lose weight, improve respiration, and increase your stamina. Start with a minimum of thirty minutes per day, four times per week. Remember, keep the pace brisk and slightly challenging—you should feel *slightly* breathless but always able to talk as you walk.

I really go to pieces at Christmas and other special occasions.

Well, don't we all? Relax. These occasions are full of family and social pressures and the appeal of traditional foods is difficult to resist. In all probability, it would *not* be a good idea to start a LifePoints weight reduction program just before the holiday season.

What should I do when I feel weak-willed and want to eat something with a very high RiskPoint number?

Eventually, your desire for such unhealthy foods will actually subside naturally on the LifePoints system, but until then why not try to choose something else. There are plenty of foods with respectable LifePoints numbers and zero or few RiskPoints. Remember, you're in control. You eat what *you* want to eat. The LifePoints system is all about taking charge of your own diet. If you want to choose bad food, then that's your decision—we're not going to nag you. But here's a tip: When you get that feeling, immediately take out a notepad, write down exactly what you want to eat, and put its RiskPoints number beside it in BIG LETTERS. Now look at what you have written. Your inclination to eat that food is sure to diminish.

I always start diets but then get fed up cooking two meals—one for myself and another for my family.

This is a difficult problem, but not an impossible one. First, sit down with your family and tell them about the LifePoints system. Then tell them that it is difficult to make two meals and that this has, in the past, caused you many problems with diets. Your family is certain to come up with a number of ideas that will help. They may even decide they want to eat healthily too.

I have always been a fast eater. When I finish my first serving, my family isn't even halfway through theirs, so I usually take another serving just to keep them company. I know this has caused a lot of my weight problems, but how can I slow down?

Here are a number of simple, unobtrusive little techniques you can use to help you eat more slowly:

- Don't cut your food into pieces all at once (if it needs cutting). Instead, cut one bite-sized piece at a time, eat it, then cut the next piece.
- Take a forkful of food, then put your fork down on the side of your plate while you chew that mouthful. Don't pick up the next forkful until you have swallowed the first.

- Buy a set of pretty cloth napkins and use one at each meal. Wipe your mouth frequently during the meal to help slow you down.
- Take a slow, deep breath in and out between mouthfuls of food. This will take the hurry out of eating and keep you relaxed as well.
- With all of this slow eating, you may think your food will go cold. Warm your plate before serving to prevent this. Also, take small portions of food so that the rest remains in the hot serving dish.

I use a lot of oil and fat in cooking and I've gotten used to the flavor. What is a good substitute for all this fat?

Cut the fat in cooking to an absolute minimum. Ignore the fat specified in the recipes you use and, when fat seems essential, try cutting the amount listed in half. Also:

- Blend a little tomato or tandoori paste with 2 ounces of water and pour this into your pan. Place over a high flame and when the liquid bubbles, add your vegetables and stir frequently. This is what we call the "new sauté" method, the liquid replacing the fat normally used in a sauté. You will be surprised at how tasty this is.
- Put the fat in serving dishes on the table instead of in your cooking. Each person can then add fat to

his own meal. If you are faced with blocks of fat
and jugs of oil, you will use very little on your food
—it just isn't appetizing.

I have a sweet tooth that always gets the better of me. What can I do to stop myself eating sweet things?

There's nothing at all wrong in eating *certain* sweet
foods. Use LifePoints to find the best. But as far as
puddings and desserts are concerned, a sweet tooth
is really a bully that always wants to have its own
way. You will have to turn it gradually into a more
respectable creature. Start by depriving your sweet
tooth, a little at a time, of what it wants. Instead of a
chocolate bar, eat some dried figs or raisins. Instead
of sugary tea or coffee, drink it unsugared with a piece
of sugarless oat cake to give you slow-release energy.
Next, try retraining your sweet tooth to become a sour
tooth. The flavors are equally strong, but the effects
are wonderfully different. Every time you want a
sweet "injection," chew on a wedge of lemon, take a
sip of cider vinegar in water, or eat a gherkin. Finally,
give yourself time to break yourself of the sweet habit.
If you have one or two bad days, don't give up. Keep
going and you will succeed.

Supercharging the System

The LifePoints system is very flexible, and can be customized to suit your individual requirements. Here are some suggestions:

- Although we suggest initially setting a maximum RiskPoints total of no more than 100 per day, this limit can be reduced if needed. For example, for a potent cholesterol-lowering regime, you might choose to observe a limit of 50 RiskPoints daily (this would ensure that you consumed no more than 20 grams of fat in your diet, only a small proportion of which would be saturated). People respond very individually to diet therapy, so a little experimentation and fine tuning might be necessary. Obviously, you should also seek the advice of your medical or health specialist in formulating an effective therapy.
- Don't make the mistake of thinking that "zero-zero" foods can be eaten abundantly. People who are used to counting calories occasionally confuse the LifePoints system with their previous dietary regime. It's not the same at all. Foods that have no RiskPoints and no LifePoints ("zero-zero") are empty foods, and have little place in your diet strategy. Remember, you have two objectives: 1) to achieve a high LifePoints score, and 2) to keep your RiskPoints within the designated limit. Zero-zero foods do *not* help you to achieve your prime dietary goal of a healthy LifePoints score. Eating a zero-zero

food is counterproductive, because it is less likely that you'll have room or the appetite to eat higher-scoring foods during the day. The LifePoints system helps you *prioritize* your food intake. Zero-zero foods have a very low priority.

....

TIP: If you eat a lot, you'll find the LifePoints Counter very helpful. Many restaurant or snack-bar foods are high in LifePoints, and low in RiskPoints, but are ruined by the addition of sauces, dressings, or other ``invisible'' supplements. With a small amount of tweaking (for example, tomato sauce instead of cream sauce on your pasta) you can eat well.

....

- Don't feel guilty about your fragmented eating habits. Today, most of us don't have the opportunity to sit down to three square meals a day; we snack when we can, and maybe eat only one "proper" meal a day. Sociologists call this "grazing," and in some respects, it mirrors our ancestral primate feeding habits. Strangely, most food and recipe books blindly fail to recognize that this is how most people actually eat. The LifePoints system is perfectly attuned to this modern way of eating, because it focuses on your *total* daily food intake. The one danger of grazing is that you consciously or subconsciously eat suboptimal food, telling yourself that you'll eat a good meal later. LifePoints can help you here, showing you how to choose the best snacks to eat. So stop feeling ashamed of your snacking, and instead, see it positively, as a new way of achieving good nutrition, with the help of the Life-Points system.

- Be aware that certain groups of the population have enhanced nutritional needs. In today's society, where food is so plentiful, it may seem strange to think that undernutrition can occur at all, but the evidence shows that it can. Although you can substantially increase your overall nutrient intake by following the LifePoints system, you should still be aware that some nutrients are not particularly easy to obtain from day-to-day food sources.

  - *Calcium:* If your dietary intake of this vital mineral is consistently too low, then bone degeneration may occur. Many people incorrectly suppose that the consumption of copious amounts of dairy produce is the only way to prevent bone-depleting afflictions such as osteoporosis. This isn't true—strangely enough, people who eat meat and dairy products are significantly more at risk of bone loss than nonmeat eaters. Good plant food sources of calcium include blackstrap molasses, sesame seeds, almonds, carob flour, tofu, and green leafy vegetables such as collards and cabbage. Calcium is best absorbed when you have adequate vitamin D in your body (sunlight is a good source) and when there's plenty of boron in the diet (available in apples and other fresh fruits and vegetables).

  - *Iron:* Since iron is well conserved by the body (90 percent of the 3 to 5 grams in our bodies is continually recycled), the major cause of iron depletion is loss of blood itself, as in menstruation. Women of childbearing years should therefore take care to eat good dietary sources of iron, which include: blackstrap molasses, pumpkin and squash seeds, many fortified breakfast cereals, quinoa, dried mixed fruit, wheat germ, and kidney beans. Foods that contain vitamin C (for example, fresh fruits and vegetables) will considerably increase your absorption. Several factors can significantly reduce the body's absorption of iron, among them tea (the tannin forms insoluble iron compounds) and the food preservative EDTA. Either of these can reduce assimilation by as much as 50 percent.

- **Vitamin B$_{12}$:** If you are eating a diet composed exclusively of plant-based foods (those from the first four groups only), then make sure you sometimes consume a good source of vitamin B$_{12}$, such as fortified breakfast cereal, fortified soya milk, yeast extract, or fermented food such as tempeh.

Now you've learned the basics of the LifePoints system. In the next chapter, we're going to explain how you can set about using it to achieve the Holy Grail of today's dieter—real, lasting weight control!

Part Two ·······························

SUCCESS BY THE INCH

• By now, you're familiar with our cheerful little motto, which we make no apology for repeating one more time: "Success by the inch is a cinch—by the yard, it's hard!" Improving your diet *one food at a time* is the real key to achieving permanent success and health. And that's precisely what the LifePoints system allows you to do. In this chapter, we'll show you how, beginning with enemy number one: fat.

Do the Fat Check

This simple quiz will probably amaze you. Devised by clever researchers at Seattle's Fred Hutchinson Cancer Research Center, it is designed to estimate the percentage of fat in your total dietary intake of calories.

You don't need to refer to anything like a food diary, so you can do it right now. Here's how: Think about your diet over the past three months and answer each of the following questions with a number from the following list. If a question doesn't apply to your diet, leave it blank. (For instance, if you don't eat red meat, don't answer questions 5, 6, and 19—your score is based on the rest of your diet.)

1 = Always
2 = Often
3 = Occasionally
4 = Rarely or never

In the past three months, when you . . .	Your answer 1 to 4
1 Ate fish, did you avoid frying it?	_____
2 Ate chicken, did you avoid frying it?	_____
3 Ate chicken, did you remove the skin?	_____
4 Ate spaghetti or noodles, did you eat it plain or with a meatless tomato sauce?	_____
5 Ate red meat, did you trim all the visible fat?	_____
6 Ate ground beef, did you choose extra lean?	_____
7 Ate bread, rolls, or muffins, did you eat them without butter or margarine?	_____
8 Drank milk, was it skim milk instead of whole?	_____
9 Ate cheese, was it a reduced-fat variety?	_____

10 Ate a frozen dessert, was it sorbet, ice milk, or
   nonfat yogurt or ice cream?   _____

11 Ate cooked vegetables, did you eat them
   without adding butter, margarine, salt pork, or
   bacon fat?   _____

12 Ate cooked vegetables, did you avoid frying
   them?   _____

13 Ate potatoes, were they cooked by a method
   other than frying?   _____

14 Ate boiled or baked potatoes, did you eat
   them without butter, margarine, or sour cream?   _____

15 Ate green salads with dressing, did you use a
   low-fat or nonfat dressing?   _____

16 Ate dessert, did you eat only fruit?   _____

17 Ate a snack, was it raw vegetables?   _____

18 Ate a snack, was it fresh fruit?   _____

19 Cooked red meat, did you trim all the fat before
   cooking?   _____

20 Used mayonnaise or a mayonnaise-type
   dressing, was it low-fat or nonfat?   _____

Now it's time to learn the truth. First, transfer the numbers above to the score sheet below, skipping any left blank. You'll see that the items are arranged within five fat-lowering strategies rather than according to their order in the quiz. Add up the total for each strategy, then whip out your calculator and follow the instructions.

Strategy 1: How well do you avoid frying your food?

Question 1 _____

Question 2 _____

Question 12 _____

Question 13 _____

Subtotal _____

Now divide by 4 to learn your average: _____

Strategy 2: How well do you avoid fatty meat?

Question 3 _____

Question 5 _____

Question 6 _____

Question 19 _____

Subtotal _____

Now divide by 4 to learn your average: _____

Strategy 3: How well do you avoid fat?

Question 4 _____

Question 7 _____

Question 11 _____

Question 14 _____

Subtotal _____

Now divide by 4 to learn your average: _____

Strategy 4: How well do you substitute low-fat or nonfat versions of foods?

Question 8 _____

Question 9 _____

Question 10 _____

Question 15 _____

Question 20 _____

Subtotal _____

Now divide by 5 to learn your average: _____

Strategy 5: How well do you replace fatty foods with fresh produce?

Question 16 _____

Question 17 _____

Question 18 _____

Subtotal _____

Now divide by 3 to learn your average: _____

Now add up all your averages and write the grand total here: _____. Finally, divide this figure by 5 to calculate your overall score, and write it here: _____. Then check the chart below:

If your overall average is	Your percentage of fat from calories is
1.0 to 1.5	under 25%
1.5 to 2	25 to 29%
2 to 2.5	30 to 34%
2.5 to 3	35 to 39%
3 to 3.5	40 to 44%
3.5 to 4	45% or more

Make sure you take the Fat Check again when you've completed your first month on the LifePoints diet.

Search and Destroy—The LifePoints Hit List

Once you've been using the LifePoint system for a few weeks, you'll begin to experiment with broadening out the range of food you eat to incorporate your own tastes, and there will, of course, be areas of change to confront as well. But for each food you decide to drop, do make sure that you introduce a new—and healthier—food to replace it. That way, improving your diet becomes a positive, sensuous experience, not a guilt-ridden exercise in personal deprivation.

••

TIP: LifePoints is not about self-denial, it's about enjoying your food—and feeling good about yourself afterward. If you really find you can't relish a meal without huge helpings of high-fat foods, try stoking up on any fresh food with a high LifePoints number before you eat your main meal. You'll find that this will significantly diminish your appetite for fats.

••

Over the next few weeks, we want you to become particularly aware of the weak spots in your diet—those aspects of your diet that one way or another deprive you of good health. In our experience, most people suffer from quite similar problem areas, which we've identified below as "targets" for you to identify and sort out.

Target Area #1

Your diet is weak if it lacks *variety*. Keep a record of the food you eat for up to one week. Include every food item and use the Counter to attribute LifePoints and RiskPoints to each food. Also, notice to which group each food belongs and tick the appropriate column. Total each column every day. Now compare the number of servings you ate from each food group to the number we suggest (see page 114). By the end of the week, you will have a pretty clear idea of what food groups you need to emphasize to achieve greater variety in your diet.

> **Destroy!** *Any overuse of groups five and six, especially at the expense of using foods from the four essential food groups.*

Target Area #2

Your diet is weak if you have one or more *meals that are always the same.* For instance, many people eat the same breakfast day in and year out. This not only means lack of variety in your diet, but it also stops you from trying new foods that will help in developing an excellent diet. If this sounds like you, make a special effort to try a new and different menu for your stuck-in-a-rut meal. Base your choices on the LifePoints Counter (pages 126–255).

> **Destroy!** *Monotony, repetitiveness, and stuck-in-a-rut habits.*

Target Area #3

Your diet is weak if you *overuse* one or more foods. For instance, many people have a tea or coffee habit that contributes to a considerable intake of full-fat milk. By the end of the day, the RiskPoints can really mount from this one food alone. Look through your daily menu to discover an overabundance of one food item. Now browse through the food listings to discover new and healthier options that will add variety and interest to your diet.

> Destroy! *Monodiets and bulk consumption of single food items.*

Target Area #4

Your diet is weak if you use too many *double-zero* foods. There are many of them around, certainly, but you don't have to eat them all. Some examples: jam, coffee, wine, sugar, most fizzy drinks, some crackers, and even a few surprises like small portions of some fruits. These foods only serve to fill you up while contributing nothing to your nutrient intake. We suggest you find alternatives to as many of them as you can. Luckily, there are many "Free Foods," which have zero RiskPoints yet offer useful numbers of LifePoints.

> Destroy! *The habits that add nothing to your LifePoints rating.*

Target Area #5

Your diet is weak if you are not eating *enough*. Does that surprise you? Many people think *diet* means *dieting,* with all the frenzy of calorie-counting that implies. Well, LifePoints, as we hope you realize by now, is different. Calories don't tell you anything about the goodness of food, so we don't use them. And calorie-counting keeps the dieter in a state of anxiety that deprives him or her of any pleasure or instinctive awareness of food. Instead, the LifePoints system uses positive information to help you achieve success and a positive attitude while creating a diet that suits you.

Destroy! *The calorie-counting frame of mind; let your diet become a positive experience rather than a worrying, punishing trial of willpower.*

When you have considered each of these five search and destroy missions, we hope you will realize that your diet is easily within your control. With ease and pleasure, you can start eating a healthy diet immediately and, as we describe below, you are probably much farther along that route than you may recognize.

Losing Weight with LifePoints

LifePoints is the world's most powerful food control system, which—unlike most other diets—does *not* sacrifice the nutritional integrity of your food for short-term weight loss. If you need to lose weight, LifePoints can help you to do so—safely, steadily, and forever. Simply follow these three steps:

1. Determine your daily RiskPoints limit. Initially, we suggest you start at a RiskPoints limit of *75 per day during weight loss,* but this limit can be adjusted to suit your individual requirements, using the table below as a guide. People respond very individually to their food, so some experimentation and fine tuning may be necessary. After the first week or so, consider revising the limit—a RiskPoints limit of 100 will ensure that your diet is still healthily low in fat, and weight loss will continue for most people.

Your RiskPoints Limit	Potential For Weight Loss
75	Provides no more than 30 grams of fat a day—the lowest suggested limit
100	Allows 40 grams of fat a day—maintains weight loss
125	Allows 50 grams of fat a day—gradual weight loss still occurs

2. Maintain your LifePoints intake. Keeping your Life-Points intake as high as you can while observing your RiskPoints limit will help to ensure that you're not sacrificing nutrition for weight loss. Your goal is to score at least 100 LifePoints every day, and more if you can, without going over your Risk-Points limit. It's not hard. To eat a healthy and varied diet, you *must* choose foods from the first four groups. Groups 5 and 6 are optional. The sug-

gested number of servings per day from each group are also listed:

Group 1	Fruit and Fruit Juices	3 servings
Group 2	Cereals, Grains, and Pasta	4 servings
Group 3	Vegetables and Vegetable Products	4 servings
Group 4	Legumes, Nuts, and Seeds	3 servings
Group 5	Meat, Fish, and Dairy	optional
Group 6	Drinks, Desserts, Snacks, and Sauces	optional

3. Follow the one-and-only rule. The LifePoints system gives you maximum freedom and doesn't hamstring you with fussy, impractical rules and instructions. Nevertheless, there's one rule you must observe: So that you eat as wide a variety of food as possible, you can only count the LifePoints for any foodstuff once, no matter how often you eat that food during the day. This means that if you eat the same food twice, only its RiskPoints count for the second helping. In other words, don't try to cheat the system by eating ten servings of broccoli for 120 LifePoints and only 10 RiskPoints! (Using this simple rule, if you ever *did* eat ten helpings of broccoli, you'd accumulate 10 RiskPoints but only 12 LifePoints.) Foods are listed in common serving sizes, but it's quite acceptable to halve or even quarter the servings, provided you similarly reduce the associated RiskPoints and LifePoints.

How does weight loss happen with LifePoints? In several natural ways. First, you'll be eating a broad and varied diet low in fat, probably much lower than you're used to. The amount and type of fat you consume is controlled by the RiskPoints number.

In addition, when you eat complex carbohydrates —which tend to be found in foods high in LifePoints —you're naturally reducing your calorie intake, without having to perform all those dreadful mental calculations. Carbohydrate-rich meals are naturally low in calories. As you may know, carbohydrates yield only 4 calories per gram, but fat provides over twice as many calories—9. So gram for gram, or ounce for ounce, carbohydrate-rich food is naturally a better deal for the slimmer.

LifePoints also helps you lose weight in another important way. By eating complex carbohydrates, you'll do something rather magical to your body's metabolic system. Here's how nutrition expert Professor Neal Barnard explains it:

Carbohydrate-rich meals are not just low in calories. They actually change your body. They readjust your hormones, which in turn boost your metabolism and speed the burning of calories. One of these hormones is the thyroid hormone. Below your Adam's apple, your thyroid gland manufactures a hormone called T4, so named because it has four iodine atoms attached. This hormone has two possible fates: It can be converted into the active form of thyroid hormone called T3, which boosts your metabolism and keeps your body burning calories, or it can be converted to an inactive hormone, called *reverse* T3. When your diet is rich in carbohydrates, more of the T4 is converted to T3, and your metabolism gets a good boost. If your diet is low in carbohydrates, more of the T4 is turned into reverse T3, resulting in a slowed metabolism. The same thing occurs during periods of very low-calorie dieting or starvation. Less of the T4 is converted to T3 and more to the useless reverse T3. This is presumably the body's way of guarding its reserves of fat; when not much food is coming in, the body conserves fat and turns down production of the fat-burning hormone T3. But a diet generous in carbohydrates keeps T3 levels high and keeps the fat fires burning.[35]

Sounds good doesn't it? But there's more. Have you ever wondered why smokers are often so thin? Perhaps you've even harbored resentful hankerings about their gaunt physiques, and wondered about taking up the weed just to trim down a bit? Well, now you can *look* like a slender smoker, without that hacking cough! As carbohydrate-rich food gradually releases sugars into the body, they stimulate the production of a neurohormone called noradrenalin, which plays an important role in instructing your body's brown fat cells (also known as brown adipose tissue) to consume stored fat. The basic function of brown fat cells is to warm the blood and distribute heat through your body, and they do this by burning fat, which is good news for slimmers. Scientists estimate that, when stimulated, brown fat can burn between 200 and 400 calories a day, which would equate to a useful weight loss of about 2 pounds a month. Smokers stimulate their brown fat cells by releasing noradrenalin into their systems. The good news is that researchers have found that the glucose released by carbohydrate-rich foods can raise your noradrenaline level by about the same amount as do cigarettes. So next time you may be tempted to reach for a coffin-nail, reach for a carrot instead.

And we're not finished yet. High LifePoints foods serve another vital function in your life: They tell you when to *stop* eating. Your body actually adjusts your appetite based on the carbohydrate content of the meals you eat. You can prove this experiment for yourself right now. First, imagine yourself with ten potato chips on a plate in front of you. Eat them. Now, do you still feel hungry? Of course you do. Actually, you would have consumed about 12 grams of fat—a significant amount. Let's do the experiment again, but this time, imagine a large baked potato in front of you. Eat it all, and ask yourself if you've still got room for more. Less likely. Both foods had the same calorie yield, but the baked potato contained a mere 0.2 grams of fat—sixty times less than the chips! If fat made you feel full, the chips would have done so. In fact, the carbohydrate-rich potato did the trick. And so will high LifePoints foods.

How much weight will you lose? Of course, this

does depend on you. Most diet books make rather outrageous claims about their potential for weight loss, yet most of them fail to back those claims up with independent scientific evidence. As a change from that, we'd like to mention some recent research that was independent, scientific, and may prove encouraging to you. In 1991, the results of the world's longest controlled human-feeding study ever to be undertaken were published. Scientifically speaking, it was a beautifully designed study.[36] Thirteen women aged between twenty-two and fifty-six were randomly put into one of two groups. The first ate a low-fat diet (at about the 125 RiskPoints limit) while the second group ate a control diet (moderately calorie-restricted but not low in fat). Both groups ate the same types of food, but the low-fat group ate reduced-fat versions (for example, low fat yogurt instead of regular). Significantly, although the low-fat group could eat as much food as they wanted to, they actually chose to consume about 250 fewer calories a day. After eleven weeks, the subjects were given a complete break for seven weeks (a so-called "washout" period) and then the tables were turned—the low-fat group went on the control diet, and the former control group ate low-fat. (This sort of study is called a "crossover" study, and is a powerful way of eliminating bias and individual idiosyncracies.) The results were very encouraging. The women on the low-fat diet had lost twice as much weight as those on the calorie-controlled diet—about half a pound a week in eleven weeks. Of course your loss may vary. This degree of weight loss may not be the fastest in the world, but it's pretty close to painless—and there's good evidence to believe that it *lasts*. As the scientists wrote:

> There is a great deal of evidence that conscious reduction in the amount of food consumed results in rapid losses of body weight; but almost invariably this lost weight is regained. Reductions in the fat content of the diet with no limitation on the amount of food consumed may lead to a more permanent weight loss than can be achieved through [conventional] dieting.

LifePoints—Beyond the Glycemic Index

How does LifePoints differ from the glycemic index, which made headlines when a spate of books on the subject of "insulin resistance" were published? "Eating Pasta Makes You Fat" trumpeted the *New York Times*. Warned another newspaper: "Contrary to current thinking, high-carbohydrate/low-fat diets are absolutely killing us."[37]

. . . .
TIP: What do you do if you've succumbed to temptation? Well, don't feel bad about it—guilt isn't going to help. Remember, with LifePoints, you can always live to fight another day, because it's a gentle process of reeducation.
. . . .

In fact, it *is* rather shocking that there should be so much fundamental confusion about what constitutes a healthy diet. The "Tufts University Diet and Nutrition Letter" made this very clear when they reviewed the book *Healthy for Life*. "What [the authors] demonstrate quite sufficiently," wrote the reviewer,

is a lack of certain basic nutrition knowledge and perspective. For instance, they call fowl, meats, and fish "high in fiber" when none of those foods contains any fiber whatsoever; it's present only in plant foods. They also imply that salads do not contain carbohydrates when in fact greens and other vegetables consist almost entirely of carbohydrates. In addition, they refer to bacon, sausage, and pastrami as "risk-reducing foods" with the rationale that those items are carbohydrate-free. And they say that more than half your calories should come from carbohydrate foods but that, if possible, carbohydrate-containing foods should be eaten only at dinner. In other words, if you eat 2,000 calories a day, you should eat more than 1,000 of them at the evening meal. To confuse matters further, they recommend that only a quarter of the food you take in at the evening meal should contain carbohydrates.[38]

Another book—dramatically entitled *The Zone*—took the glycemic index theory still farther. The author argued that the proportion of protein to carbohydrate you eat determines the eicosanoids your body produces. Eicosanoids? Well, they're hormonelike substances that include prostaglandins, leukotrienes, and thromboxanes. If you eat a "40-30-30" diet—in other words, 40 percent of your calories as carbohydrates, 30 percent as protein, and 30 percent as fat—you're supposed to be able to control those rogue eicosanoids, and so conquer your weight, your susceptibility to diseases, your mood, and your physical performance. But what evidence is there for these claims? Precious little. Comments William Evans, Ph.D., director of the Noll Physiological Research Center at Penn State University: "Eicosanoids are metabolism by-products, but they're not the gates to disease. There aren't any studies that I'm familiar with that suggest they're dangerous in any way. Anyone who tries to sell diet as the key to stemming "bad" eicosanoid production is capitalizing on an unfounded idea."[39]

Do we *really* need to create yet another nutritional enemy—in this case, insulin or eicosanoids? While it's true that insulin plays an important role in fat metabolism, where is the scientific *evidence* that eating carbohydrates can cause insulin-related weight gain? So far, it simply hasn't been presented, which is rather strange for such an allegedly revolutionary theory. In fact, many good studies have shown exactly the opposite—that switching to a high-carbohydrate, low-fat diet will indeed lead to worthwhile weight loss.

So is there *any* use for the glycemic index? In fact, there is. The concept was first proposed by German scientists back in 1973, when they noted that various carbohydrate foodstuffs produced different blood sugar responses in individuals.[40] Before then, all scientists had assumed that complex carbohydrates (for example, wheat) were healthier for diabetics than simple carbohydrates (for example, sugar). Unfortunately, this simple proposition had never actually been put to the test.[41] When it was, conventional wisdom seemed to be overturned—for example, the kind of sugar found in fruit (fructose) was given a glycemic index of 30, table sugar rated 86, and white bread 100. This meant that white bread is worse than fruit sugar in terms of glucose control for diabetics.

So for diabetics, the glycemic index *might* be a useful guide for estimating the likely effect of various foods on their blood sugar level. However, even here there are some significant problems. The index is calculated in the laboratory, using human subjects, who are fed a test food and then have six blood samples taken from them over two hours. The blood is then analyzed and the results computed to produce a number—the glycemic index. It all sounds very neat and tidy, but in the real world things aren't nearly so simple:

- Humans differ *very* considerably in their response to food: the same food item, when eaten by different people, can produce a fourfold variation in glycemic response.[42]

em in quite the same way again. We hope you
he thrill we first felt when we realized just how
ve and uncomplicated the LifePoints system is to
eer power over your diet—at your fingertips!

oints Food Group One:
and Fruit Juices

	Measure	X Risk-Points	✓ Life-Points
A			
NDIAN			
)	juice (1 CUP 242G)	1	10
	raw (1 CUP 98G)	0	9
	baked with sugar, flesh, and skin (1 FRUIT 138G)	0	2
	canned, sweetened (1 CUP SLICES 204G)	2	1
	dehydrated (low moisture) uncooked (1 CUP 60G)	0	3
	dried sulfured uncooked (1 CUP 86G)	0	4
	juice canned or bottled w/added vitamin C (1 CUP 248G)	0	3
	juice canned or bottled wo/added vitamin C (1 CUP 248G)	0	1
	juice frozen concentrated, diluted w/3 vol water w/added vitamin C (1 CUP 239G)	0	2

- The method of preparing or cooking the food can greatly alter the food's glycemic index. In particular, the particle size of the food (for example, if it's puréed) can make a considerable difference to the body's blood sugar response, and hence to the glycemic index.[43]
- Even within the same food, different strains can produce very different results. For example, new potatoes have a glycemic index of 80, but russet potatoes are 116—nearly 50 percent higher!
- The glycemic index is calculated by feeding people one food at a time. But outside of the laboratory, people don't eat like that. For example, a fatty meal will lengthen the time food takes to pass through the upper gastrointestinal tract, and so produce a lower glycemic response. Protein, on the other hand, will increase the body's insulin secretion, leading to more rapid glucose processing.[44]

Taking all this into account, what use is the glycemic index for the rest of us? Well, choosing your diet solely on the basis of a food's glycemic index is plain silly—there are far too many uncertainties associated with it, not the least of which would be the fact that you'd end up eating a diet far too high in fat. And if you're concerned about the possible impact of carbohydrates on your insulin secretion—and hence on your weight control—here's a tip: Try snacking! Changing the way you eat your food can have a very profound effect on insulin levels. When scientists fed two groups of volunteers either three meals or seventeen snacks every day, they were amazed to find that the people who snacked frequently had lowered their cholesterol by 15 percent and slashed their average blood insulin levels by nearly 28 percent. If you choose to try this, you must ensure that you're eating healthy snacks.

Part Three · · · · · · · · · · · ·

THE LIFEPOINTS COUNTER

▪ LifePoints is all about freedom—the according to your own personal tastes to the likes or dislikes of diet book why at the heart of the LifePoints counter—a unique listing of foods major groups (remember, the first f sory, the last two optional). The Life trol system is very powerful, and number of ways. For example, you lyze your existing diet, and see wh You can use it to plan a really hea the guidelines explained in Part T —the easiest way of all—you car tem to check out the difference to find the healthiest. One thir glance through the foods that

view
share
effect
use.

Life
Fru

Food
· · · · · ·
ACER
(WEST
CHER

APPLE

Food	Measure	X Risk-Points	✓ Life-Points
	raw w/skin (1 FRUIT 3/LB 138G)	1	1
	raw wo/skin (1 FRUIT 3/LB 128G)	0	1
APPLESAUCE	canned sweetened (1 CUP 255G)	1	2
	canned unsweetened (1 CUP 244G)	0	2
APRICOT	canned (1 CUP HALVES 258G)	0	4
	dehydrated (low moisture) stewed (1 CUP 249G)	1	13
	dehydrated (low moisture) uncooked (1 CUP 119G)	1	16
	dried stewed w/added sugar (1 CUP HALVES 270G)	1	7
	dried stewed wo/added sugar (1 CUP HALVES 250G)	1	9
	dried uncooked (1 CUP HALVES 130G)	1	14
	juice canned w/added vitamin C (1 CUP 251G)	0	4
	raw (3 FRUITS 12/LB 106G)	1	3
AVOCADO	raw (1 CUP PURÉE 230G)	88	21
	raw (1 FRUIT WO/SKIN AND SEEDS 201G)	76	18
BANANA	dehydrated or banana powder (1 CUP 100G)	5	7
	raw (1 CUP MASHED 225G)	3	13
	raw (1 FRUIT WO/SKIN AND SEEDS 114G)	1	6

Food	Measure	Risk-Points	Life-Points
BLACKBERRY	canned solids and liquid (1 CUP 256G)	0	9
	raw (1 CUP 144G)	1	6
BLUEBERRY	canned solids and liquid (1 CUP 256G)	2	3
	frozen (1 CUP THAWED 230G)	0	4
	raw (1 CUP 145G)	1	3
BOYSENBERRY	canned (1 CUP 256G)	0	9
CARAMBOLA (STARFRUIT)	raw (1 FRUIT WO/SEEDS 127G)	1	2
CHERIMOYA	raw (½ FRUIT WITHOUT SKIN AND SEEDS 273G)	2	8
CHERRY	pie filling (½ CUP 125G)	0	3
	sour red canned (1 CUP 256G)	0	5
	sour red raw (1 CUP WO/PITS 155G)	1	3
	stewed (1 CUP 250G)	0	2
	sweet canned (1 CUP WO/PITS 257G)	0	4
	sweet raw (1 CUP 145G)	3	3
CLEMENTINE	whole (1 FRUIT 100G)	0	3
CRANBERRY	juice cocktail (1 CUP 253G)	0	2
	sauce canned (1 CUP 277G)	1	2
	and orange relish (1 CUP 275G)	0	2
CURRANT	European black raw (1 CUP 112G)	1	5

Food	Measure	Risk-Points ✗	Life-Points ✓
	red and white raw (1 CUP 112G)	0	3
DAMSON PLUM	raw (1 CUP SLICES 165G)	0	4
	raw (1 FRUIT 66G)	0	1
	stewed (3 FRUIT 133G)	0	2
DATE	domestic natural and dry (1 CUP CHOPPED 178G)	2	11
ELDERBERRY	raw (1 CUP 145G)	1	7
FIG	canned (1 CUP 259G)	0	3
	dried stewed (1 CUP 259G)	3	10
	dried uncooked (1 CUP 199G)	5	15
	raw (1 LRG FRUIT WO/STEM 64G)	0	1
FRUIT COCKTAIL	(peach, pineapple, pear, grape, and cherry) canned (1 CUP 255G)	0	3
	(peach, pear, and pineapple) canned (1 CUP 255G)	0	5
FRUIT SALAD	homemade (½ CUP 128G)	0	3
GOOSEBERRY	canned (1 CUP 252G)	1	4
GRAPE	American type (slip skin) raw (1 CUP 92G)	0	2
	European type (adherent skin) raw (1 CUP 160G)	2	4
	juice canned or bottled (1 CUP 253G)	0	3
	juice frozen concentrate diluted w/3 vol water (1 CUP 250G)	0	2

Food	Measure	Risk-Points ✗	Life-Points ✓
GRAPEFRUIT	juice canned (1 CUP 250G)	0	4
	juice raw (1 CUP 247G)	0	5
	raw pink and red all areas (1 CUP SECTIONS W/JUICE 230G)	0	4
GREENGAGE PLUM	raw (1 FRUIT 66G)	0	1
GROUND-CHERRY	raw (1 CUP 140G)	2	5
GUAVA	canned (1 CUP 165G)	0	7
	sauce cooked (1 CUP 238G)	0	7
JUJUBE (CHINESE DATE)	dried (1 SERVING 100G)	2	6
	raw (1 SERVING 100G)	0	2
KIWIFRUIT (CHINESE GOOSEBERRIES)	fresh raw (1 MED FRUIT WO/SKIN 76G)	0	2
KUMQUAT	raw (1 FRUIT 19G)	0	0
LEMON	juice canned, bottled, or raw (1 CUP 244G)	0	5
	juice canned, bottled, or raw (1 TBSP 15G)	0	0
	peel raw (1 TBSP 6G)	0	0
	raw wo/peel (1 MED FRUIT 58G)	0	1
LIME	juice canned, bottled, or raw (1 CUP 246G)	0	3

Food	Measure	✗ Risk-Points	✓ Life-Points
	juice canned, bottled, or raw (1 TBSP 15G)	0	0
LONGAN	dried (1 SERVING 100G)	1	8
	raw (1 SERVING 100G)	0	2
LOQUAT (JAPONICA)	raw (1 CUP 190G)	0	2
LYCHEE	canned in syrup (½ CUP 130G)	0	1
	dried (1 SERVING 100G)	3	10
	raw (1 CUP 190G)	2	4
MAMMY-APPLE (MAMEY)	raw (½ FRUIT 423G)	5	7
MANGO	juice, canned (1 CUP 251G)	1	3
	raw (1 CUP SLICES 165G)	1	5
	raw (1 FRUIT 207G)	1	7
MELON	balls frozen (1 CUP 173G)	1	7
	cantaloupe raw (1 CUP CUBED PIECES 160G)	1	6
	cantaloupe raw (½ FRUIT 5" DIAM 267G)	1	10
	casaba raw (1 CUP CUBED PIECES 170G)	0	2
	honeydew raw (1 CUP CUBED PIECES 170G)	0	3
	honeydew raw (¹⁄₁₀ FRUIT 129G)	0	2
MIXED FRUIT	dried (1 HANDFUL 60G)	0	3

Food	Measure	✗ Risk-Points	✓ Life-Points
NECTARINE	raw (1 CUP SLICES 138G)	1	2
OLIVE	ripe canned (1 LARGE 4G)	1	0
	ripe canned (super colossal) (1 SUPER COLOSSAL 15G)	2	0
ORANGE	juice canned (1 CUP 249G)	0	7
	juice raw (1 CUP 248G)	1	9
	juice raw (JUICE FROM 1 FRUIT 86G)	0	3
	peel raw (1 TBSP 6G)	0	0
	raw all commercial varieties (1 FRUIT 2⅜" DIAM 131G)	0	6
	raw w/peel (1 FRUIT 159G)	1	7
	and grapefruit juice canned (1 CUP 247G)	0	6
PAPAYA	nectar canned (1 CUP 250G)	0	2
	raw (1 FRUIT 304G)	1	12
PASSION FRUIT (GRANADILLA)	purple raw (1 FRUIT 18G)	0	0
	juice purple raw (1 CUP 247G)	0	5
	juice yellow raw (1 CUP 247G)	1	7
PEACH	canned solids and liquid (1 CUP HALVES OR SLICES 256G)	0	3
	dehydrated (low moisture) stewed (1 CUP 242G)	2	9

- The method of preparing or cooking the food can greatly alter the food's glycemic index. In particular, the particle size of the food (for example, if it's puréed) can make a considerable difference to the body's blood sugar response, and hence to the glycemic index.[43]
- Even within the same food, different strains can produce very different results. For example, new potatoes have a glycemic index of 80, but russet potatoes are 116—nearly 50 percent higher!
- The glycemic index is calculated by feeding people one food at a time. But outside of the laboratory, people don't eat like that. For example, a fatty meal will lengthen the time food takes to pass through the upper gastrointestinal tract, and so produce a lower glycemic response. Protein, on the other hand, will increase the body's insulin secretion, leading to more rapid glucose processing.[44]

Taking all this into account, what use is the glycemic index for the rest of us? Well, choosing your diet solely on the basis of a food's glycemic index is plain silly—there are far too many uncertainties associated with it, not the least of which would be the fact that you'd end up eating a diet far too high in fat. And if you're concerned about the possible impact of carbohydrates on your insulin secretion—and hence on your weight control—here's a tip: Try snacking! Changing the way you eat your food can have a very profound effect on insulin levels. When scientists fed two groups of volunteers either three meals or seventeen snacks every day, they were amazed to find that the people who snacked frequently had lowered their cholesterol by 15 percent and slashed their average blood insulin levels by nearly 28 percent. If you choose to try this, you must ensure that you're eating healthy snacks.

Part Three ·······················

THE LIFEPOINTS COUNTER

• LifePoints is all about freedom—the freedom to eat according to your own personal tastes, not according to the likes or dislikes of diet book authors. That's why at the heart of the LifePoints system lies the counter—a unique listing of foods divided into six major groups (remember, the first four are compulsory, the last two optional). The LifePoints food control system is very powerful, and can be used in a number of ways. For example, you can use it to analyze your existing diet, and see where the holes are. You can use it to plan a really healthy diet, following the guidelines explained in Part Two of this book. Or —the easiest way of all—you can simply use the system to check out the difference between two foods, to find the healthiest. One thing is certain: As you glance through the foods that follow, you'll never view them in quite the same way again. We hope you share the thrill we first felt when we realized just how effective and uncomplicated the LifePoints system is to use. Sheer power over your diet—at your fingertips!

LifePoints Food Group One: Fruit and Fruit Juices

Food	Measure	✗ Risk-Points	✓ Life-Points
ACEROLA (WEST INDIAN CHERRY)	juice (1 CUP 242G)	1	10
	raw (1 CUP 98G)	0	9
APPLE	baked with sugar, flesh, and skin (1 FRUIT 138G)	0	2
	canned, sweetened (1 CUP SLICES 204G)	2	1
	dehydrated (low moisture) uncooked (1 CUP 60G)	0	3
	dried sulfured uncooked (1 CUP 86G)	0	4
	juice canned or bottled w/added vitamin C (1 CUP 248G)	0	3
	juice canned or bottled wo/added vitamin C (1 CUP 248G)	0	1
	juice frozen concentrated, diluted w/3 vol water w/added vitamin C (1 CUP 239G)	0	2

Food	Measure	✗ Risk-Points	✓ Life-Points
	raw w/skin (1 FRUIT 3/LB 138G)	1	1
	raw wo/skin (1 FRUIT 3/LB 128G)	0	1
APPLESAUCE	canned sweetened (1 CUP 255G)	1	2
	canned unsweetened (1 CUP 244G)	0	2
APRICOT	canned (1 CUP HALVES 258G)	0	4
	dehydrated (low moisture) stewed (1 CUP 249G)	1	13
	dehydrated (low moisture) uncooked (1 CUP 119G)	1	16
	dried stewed w/added sugar (1 CUP HALVES 270G)	1	7
	dried stewed wo/added sugar (1 CUP HALVES 250G)	1	9
	dried uncooked (1 CUP HALVES 130G)	1	14
	juice canned w/added vitamin C (1 CUP 251G)	0	4
	raw (3 FRUITS 12/LB 106G)	1	3
AVOCADO	raw (1 CUP PURÉE 230G)	88	21
	raw (1 FRUIT WO/SKIN AND SEEDS 201G)	76	18
BANANA	dehydrated or banana powder (1 CUP 100G)	5	7
	raw (1 CUP MASHED 225G)	3	13
	raw (1 FRUIT WO/SKIN AND SEEDS 114G)	1	6

Food	Measure	Risk-Points	Life-Points
BLACKBERRY	canned solids and liquid (1 CUP 256G)	0	9
	raw (1 CUP 144G)	1	6
BLUEBERRY	canned solids and liquid (1 CUP 256G)	2	3
	frozen (1 CUP THAWED 230G)	0	4
	raw (1 CUP 145G)	1	3
BOYSENBERRY	canned (1 CUP 256G)	0	9
CARAMBOLA (STARFRUIT)	raw (1 FRUIT WO/SEEDS 127G)	1	2
CHERIMOYA	raw (½ FRUIT WITHOUT SKIN AND SEEDS 273G)	2	8
CHERRY	pie filling (½ CUP 125G)	0	3
	sour red canned (1 CUP 256G)	0	5
	sour red raw (1 CUP WO/PITS 155G)	1	3
	stewed (1 CUP 250G)	0	2
	sweet canned (1 CUP WO/PITS 257G)	0	4
	sweet raw (1 CUP 145G)	3	3
CLEMENTINE	whole (1 FRUIT 100G)	0	3
CRANBERRY	juice cocktail (1 CUP 253G)	0	2
	sauce canned (1 CUP 277G)	1	2
	and orange relish (1 CUP 275G)	0	2
CURRANT	European black raw (1 CUP 112G)	1	5

Food	Measure	X Risk-Points	✓ Life-Points
	red and white raw (1 CUP 112G)	0	3
DAMSON PLUM	raw (1 CUP SLICES 165G)	0	4
	raw (1 FRUIT 66G)	0	1
	stewed (3 FRUIT 133G)	0	2
DATE	domestic natural and dry (1 CUP CHOPPED 178G)	2	11
ELDERBERRY	raw (1 CUP 145G)	1	7
FIG	canned (1 CUP 259G)	0	3
	dried stewed (1 CUP 259G)	3	10
	dried uncooked (1 CUP 199G)	5	15
	raw (1 LRG FRUIT WO/STEM 64G)	0	1
FRUIT COCKTAIL	(peach, pineapple, pear, grape, and cherry) canned (1 CUP 255G)	0	3
	(peach, pear, and pineapple) canned (1 CUP 255G)	0	5
FRUIT SALAD	homemade (½ CUP 128G)	0	3
GOOSEBERRY	canned (1 CUP 252G)	1	4
GRAPE	American type (slip skin) raw (1 CUP 92G)	0	2
	European type (adherent skin) raw (1 CUP 160G)	2	4
	juice canned or bottled (1 CUP 253G)	0	3
	juice frozen concentrate diluted w/3 vol water (1 CUP 250G)	0	2

Food	Measure	✗ Risk-Points	✓ Life-Points
GRAPEFRUIT	juice canned (1 CUP 250G)	0	4
	juice raw (1 CUP 247G)	0	5
	raw pink and red all areas (1 CUP SECTIONS W/JUICE 230G)	0	4
GREENGAGE PLUM	raw (1 FRUIT 66G)	0	1
GROUND-CHERRY	raw (1 CUP 140G)	2	5
GUAVA	canned (1 CUP 165G)	0	7
	sauce cooked (1 CUP 238G)	0	7
JUJUBE (CHINESE DATE)	dried (1 SERVING 100G)	2	6
	raw (1 SERVING 100G)	0	2
KIWIFRUIT (CHINESE GOOSEBERRIES)	fresh raw (1 MED FRUIT WO/SKIN 76G)	0	2
KUMQUAT	raw (1 FRUIT 19G)	0	0
LEMON	juice canned, bottled, or raw (1 CUP 244G)	0	5
	juice canned, bottled, or raw (1 TBSP 15G)	0	0
	peel raw (1 TBSP 6G)	0	0
	raw wo/peel (1 MED FRUIT 58G)	0	1
LIME	juice canned, bottled, or raw (1 CUP 246G)	0	3

Food	Measure	✗ Risk-Points	✓ Life-Points
	juice canned, bottled, or raw (1 TBSP 15G)	0	0
LONGAN	dried (1 SERVING 100G)	1	8
	raw (1 SERVING 100G)	0	2
LOQUAT (JAPONICA)	raw (1 CUP 190G)	0	2
LYCHEE	canned in syrup (½ CUP 130G)	0	1
	dried (1 SERVING 100G)	3	10
	raw (1 CUP 190G)	2	4
MAMMY-APPLE (MAMEY)	raw (½ FRUIT 423G)	5	7
MANGO	juice, canned (1 CUP 251G)	1	3
	raw (1 CUP SLICES 165G)	1	5
	raw (1 FRUIT 207G)	1	7
MELON	balls frozen (1 CUP 173G)	1	7
	cantaloupe raw (1 CUP CUBED PIECES 160G)	1	6
	cantaloupe raw (½ FRUIT 5" DIAM 267G)	1	10
	casaba raw (1 CUP CUBED PIECES 170G)	0	2
	honeydew raw (1 CUP CUBED PIECES 170G)	0	3
	honeydew raw (1/10 FRUIT 129G)	0	2
MIXED FRUIT	dried (1 HANDFUL 60G)	0	3

Food	Measure	X Risk-Points	✓ Life-Points
NECTARINE	raw (1 CUP SLICES 138G)	1	2
OLIVE	ripe canned (1 LARGE 4G)	1	0
	ripe canned (super colossal) (1 SUPER COLOSSAL 15G)	2	0
ORANGE	juice canned (1 CUP 249G)	0	7
	juice raw (1 CUP 248G)	1	9
	juice raw (JUICE FROM 1 FRUIT 86G)	0	3
	peel raw (1 TBSP 6G)	0	0
	raw all commercial varieties (1 FRUIT 2⅜" DIAM 131G)	0	6
	raw w/peel (1 FRUIT 159G)	1	7
	and grapefruit juice canned (1 CUP 247G)	0	6
PAPAYA	nectar canned (1 CUP 250G)	0	2
	raw (1 FRUIT 304G)	1	12
PASSION FRUIT (GRANADILLA)	purple raw (1 FRUIT 18G)	0	0
	juice purple raw (1 CUP 247G)	0	5
	juice yellow raw (1 CUP 247G)	1	7
PEACH	canned solids and liquid (1 CUP HALVES OR SLICES 256G)	0	3
	dehydrated (low moisture) stewed (1 CUP 242G)	2	9

Food	Measure	✗ Risk-Points	✓ Life-Points
	dehydrated (low moisture) uncooked (1 CUP 116G)	2	10
	dried stewed (1 CUP HALVES 270G)	1	6
	dried uncooked (1 CUP HALVES 160G)	3	14
	nectar canned (1 CUP 249G)	0	2
	raw (1 CUP SLICE 170G)	0	3
	raw (1 FRUIT 4/LB 87G)	0	1
PEAR	Asian (Chinese) raw (1 FRUIT 122G)	0	1
	canned solids and liquid (1 CUP HALVES 255G)	0	2
	dried stewed (1 CUP HALVES 280G)	2	6
	dried uncooked (1 CUP HALVES 180G)	2	9
	nectar canned (1 CUP 250G)	0	2
	raw (1 CUP SLICES 165G)	1	2
	raw (1 FRUIT 2.5/LB 166G)	1	2
PERSIMMON	Japanese dried (1 FRUIT 34G)	0	1
	Japanese raw (1 FRUIT 2½" DIAM 168G)	0	3
	native raw (1 FRUIT 25G)	0	0
PINEAPPLE	canned solids and liquid (1 CUP CHUNKS CRUSHED 255G)	0	5
	juice canned (1 CUP 250G)	0	8
	raw (1 CUP DICED PIECES 155G)	1	4

Food	Measure	Risk-Points	Life-Points
	raw (1 SLICE 3½" DIAM 84G)	0	2
PLANTAIN	cooked (1 CUP SLICES 154G)	0	7
	raw (1 FRUIT 179G)	1	9
PLUM	canned purple solids and liquid (1 CUP 258G)	0	4
	raw (1 CUP SLICES 165G)	2	3
	raw (1 FRUIT 2⅛" DIAM 66G)	1	1
	stewed (3 FRUIT 133G)	0	2
POMEGRANATE	juice fresh (1 CUP 251G)	0	5
	raw (1 FRUIT 3⅜" DIAM 154G)	1	2
PRUNE	canned solids and liquid (1 CUP 234G)	1	9
	dehydrated (low moisture) stewed (1 CUP 280G)	1	9
	dehydrated (low moisture) uncooked (1 CUP 132G)	2	14
	dried stewed (1 CUP WO/PITS 212G)	1	9
	dried uncooked (1 CUP WO/PITS 161G)	2	13
	juice canned (1 CUP 256G)	0	8
RAISIN	golden seedless (1 CUP NOT PACKED 145G)	1	9
	seedless (1 CUP NOT PACKED 145G)	1	9
RASPBERRY	canned red solids and liquid (1 CUP 256G)	0	6

Food	Measure	X Risk-Points	✓ Life-Points
	frozen red (1 CUP 250G)	1	9
	raw (1 CUP 123G)	1	6
	stewed (½ CUP 128G)	0	3
RHUBARB	cooked w/sugar (1 CUP 240G)	0	6
SHARON FRUIT	raw (1 FRUIT 56G)	0	1
SOURSOP	raw (1 CUP PULP 225G)	1	6
STRAWBERRY	frozen whole (1 CUP 255G)	0	5
	raw (1 CUP 149G)	1	5
TAMARIND	raw (1 CUP PULP 120G)	2	10
TANGERINE	juice canned or raw (1 CUP 249G)	1	4
	mandarin orange, canned (1 CUP 249G)	0	7
	mandarin orange, raw (1 CUP SECTIONS 195G)	0	7
WATERMELON	raw (1 CUP DICED PIECES 160G)	1	3

LifePoints Food Group Two: Cereals, Grains, and Pasta

Breakfast Cereals

The average weight of most servings of breakfast cereals is about an ounce: First choose your cereal, then add milk as on page 140. You should be aware that many breakfast cereals have high LifePoints ratings because they are fortified by the manufacturers with vitamins, which means that they are not strictly comparable to other, unfortified foods.

Food	Measure	X Risk-Points	✓ Life-Points
100% BRAN	(wheat bran barley) (1 OZ 28G)	3	32
40% BRAN FLAKES	Kellogg's (wheat bran) (1 OZ 28G)	1	33
	Post (wheat bran) (1 OZ 28G)	1	26
	Ralston Purina (wheat bran) (1 OZ 28G)	0	26
ALL-BRAN	(wheat bran) (1 OZ 28G)	1	23
ALPHA-BITS	oat with other grains (1 OZ 28G)	1	24
APPLE JACKS	corn with other grains (1 OZ 28G)	0	21
BRAN BUDS	wheat bran (1 OZ 28G)	1	23
BRAN CHEX	wheat bran and corn (1 OZ 28G)	1	24
CAP'N CRUNCH	(corn with other grains) (1 OZ 28G)	12	34
	crunchberries (corn oat) (1 OZ 28G)	11	32
	peanut butter (corn with other grains) (1 OZ 28G)	11	35
CHEERIOS	(oat and wheat) (1 OZ 28G)	4	21
COCOA KRISPIES	(rice) (1 OZ 28G)	0	18
COCOA PEBBLES	(rice) (1 OZ 28G)	3	24

Food	Measure	✗ Risk-Points	✓ Life-Points
COOKIE CRISP	choc chip and vanilla (corn with other grains) (1 OZ 28G)	2	19
CORN BRAN	(corn bran with other grains) (1 OZ 28G)	2	33
CORN CHEX	(corn) (1 OZ 28G)	0	20
CORN FLAKES	Kellogg's (corn) (1 OZ 28G)	0	17
	low sodium (corn) (1 OZ 28G)	0	1
CRISP RICE	low sodium (rice) (1 OZ 28G)	0	2
CRISPY RICE	(rice) (1 OZ 28G)	0	3
CRISPY WHEATS 'N RAISINS	(wheat) (1 OZ 28G)	1	20
FORTIFIED OAT FLAKES	(oat with other grains) (1 OZ 28G)	1	28
FROOT LOOPS	(corn with other grains) (1 OZ 28G)	1	21
FROSTED MINI-WHEATS	(bite-sized wheat) (1 OZ 28G)	0	19
FROSTED RICE KRINKLES	(rice) (1 OZ 28G)	0	24
FROSTED RICE KRISPIES	(rice) (1 OZ 28G)	0	17
FRUITY PEBBLES	(rice) (1 OZ 28G)	3	24
GOLDEN GRAHAMS	(corn wheat) (1 OZ 28G)	5	20
GRAHAM CRACKOS	(wheat) (1 OZ 28G)	0	18

Food	Measure	Risk-Points ✗	Life-Points ✓
GRANOLA	homemade (oats, wheat germ) (1 OZ 28G)	19	5
GRAPE-NUTS	flakes (wheat barley) (1 OZ 28G)	0	27
	(wheat barley) (1 OZ 28G)	0	23
HONEY NUT CHEERIOS	(oat, wheat) (1 OZ 28G)	1	21
HONEY AND NUT CORN FLAKES	(corn) (1 OZ 28G)	3	17
HONEYBRAN	(wheat) (1 OZ 28G)	1	21
HONEYCOMB	(corn, oats) (1 OZ 28G)	1	24
KIX	(corn with other grains) (1 OZ 28G)	1	27
LIFE	plain and cinnamon products (oat with other grains) (1 OZ 28G)	1	19
LUCKY CHARMS	(oat with other grains) (1 OZ 28G)	2	20
MALTEX	cooked with water (wheat) (¾ CUP 187G)	1	6
	dry (wheat) (1 CUP 151G)	7	26
MAYPO	cooked with water with salt (oats with other grains) (¾ CUP 180G)	4	29
	cooked with water without salt (oats with other grains) (¾ CUP 180G)	4	29
	dry (oats with other grains) (1 CUP 94G)	12	59
MOST	(wheat bran, wheat) (1 OZ 28G)	0	60

Food	Measure	✗ Risk-Points	✓ Life-Points
NUTRI-GRAIN	barley (barley) (1 OZ 28G)	0	25
	corn (corn) (1 OZ 28G)	1	25
	rye (rye) (1 OZ 28G)	0	25
	wheat (wheat) (1 OZ 28G)	0	25
PRODUCT 19	(corn with other grains) (1 OZ 28G)	0	59
RAISIN BRAN	Kellogg's (wheat) (1 OZ 28G)	1	26
	Post (wheat) (1 OZ 28G)	1	26
	Ralston Purina (wheat) (1 OZ 28G)	0	25
RAISINS RICE & RYE	(rice with other grains) (1 OZ 28G)	0	21
RICE CHEX	(rice) (1 OZ 28G)	0	20
RICE KRISPIES	(rice) (1 OZ 28G)	0	17
RICE, PUFFED	fortified (rice) (1 OZ 28G)	0	18
	lower fortification (<2% RDA) (rice) (1 OZ 28G)	0	1
SPECIAL K	(rice wheat) (1 OZ 28G)	0	22
SUGAR CORN POPS	(corn) (1 OZ 28G)	0	18
SUGAR FROSTED FLAKES	Kellogg's (corn) (1 OZ 28G)	0	17
	Ralston Purina (corn) (1 OZ 28G)	0	18
SUGAR SMACKS	(wheat) (1 OZ 28G)	1	17

Food	Measure	Risk-Points	Life-Points
SUGAR SPARKLED FLAKES	(corn) (1 OZ 28G)	0	22
SUPER SUGAR CRISP	(wheat) (1 OZ 28G)	0	24
TEAM	(rice with other grains) (1 OZ 28G)	1	18
TOASTIES	(corn) (1 OZ 28G)	0	22
TOTAL	(wheat) (1 OZ 28G)	1	61
TRIX	(corn with other grains) (1 OZ 28G)	0	19
WAFFELOS	(wheat with other grains) (1 OZ 28G)	2	19
WHEAT CHEX	(wheat) (1 OZ 28G)	1	23
WHEAT 'N RAISIN CHEX	(wheat) (1 OZ 28G)	0	19
WHEAT, PUFFED	fortified (rice) (1 OZ 28G)	0	19
	lower fortification (<2% RDA) (wheat) (1 OZ 28G)	0	5
WHEAT, SHREDDED	large biscuit (wheat) (2 ROUND BISCUITS 38G)	1	6
	small biscuit (wheat) (1 OZ 28G)	1	5
WHEATIES	(wheat) (1 OZ 28G)	1	26
MILK: COW'S	virtually fat free (¾ CUP 183G)	0	9
	semiskimmed (¾ CUP 183G)	13	10
	skimmed (¾ CUP 183G)	1	9

Food	Measure	X Risk-Points	✓ Life-Points
	whole (¾ CUP 183G)	32	9
MILK: GOAT	(¾ CUP 183G)	36	7
MILK: SOYA	(¾ CUP 183G)	8	5

COOKED BREAKFAST FOODS

Food	Measure	X Risk-Points	✓ Life-Points
CORN GRITS	instant plain prepared with water (corn) (1 PKT PREPARED 137G)	0	3
	instant with artificial cheese flavor prepared with water (corn) (1 PKT PREPARED 142G)	2	4
	instant with imitation bacon bits prepared with water (corn) (1 PKT PREPARED 141G)	1	4
	instant with imitation ham bits prepared with water (corn soy) (1 PKT PREPARED 141G)	1	5
	white regular and quick enriched cooked with water (corn) (¾ CUP 182G)	0	4
	white regular and quick unenriched cooked with water (corn) (¾ CUP 182G)	0	1
	yellow regular and quick enriched cooked with water (corn) (¾ CUP 182G)	0	4

Food	Measure	Risk-Points ✗	Life-Points ✓
	yellow regular and quick unenriched cooked with water (corn) (¾ CUP 182G)	0	1
CREAM OF RICE	cooked with water (rice) (¾ CUP 183G)	0	1
CREAM OF WHEAT	instant prepared with water (wheat) (¾ CUP 181G)	0	8
	mix'n eat apple, banana, and maple flavor prepared (wheat corn) (1 PKT PREPARED 150G)	1	20
	mix'n eat plain prepared with water (wheat corn) (1 PKT PREPARED 142G)	0	20
	quick cooked with water (wheat) (¾ CUP 179G)	0	7
	regular cooked with water (wheat) (¾ CUP 188G)	0	7
FARINA	enriched cooked with water (wheat) (¾ CUP 175G)	0	3
	unenriched cooked with water (wheat) (¾ CUP 175G)	0	1
OATS	instant fortified plain prepared with water (oats) (1 PKT PREPARED 177G)	4	27
	instant fortified with apples and cinnamon prepared with water (oats) (1 PKT PREPARED 149G)	4	24

Food	Measure	✗ Risk-Points	✓ Life-Points
	instant fortified with bran and raisins prepared with water (oats wheat bran) (1 PKT PREPARED 195G)	4	31
	instant fortified with cinnamon and spice prepared with water (oats) (1 PKT PREPARED 161G)	4	28
	instant fortified with maple and brown sugar flavor prepared with water (oats) (1 PKT PREPARED 155G)	4	26
	instant fortified with raisins and spice prepared with water (oats) (1 PKT PREPARED 158G)	4	27
	regular, quick, and instant without fortification cooked with water (oats) (¾ CUP 175G)	4	4
	Ralston cooked with water (oats) (¾ CUP 190G)	1	6
ROMAN MEAL	plain cooked with water (wheat with other grains) (¾ CUP 181G)	1	6
	with oats cooked with water (wheat with other grains) (¾ CUP 180G)	3	8
WAFFLES	buttermilk prepared from recipe (1 WAFFLE 75G)	25	8
	frozen ready-to-heat toasted (includes buttermilk) (1 WAFFLE 33G)	6	9
	plain prepared from recipe (1 WAFFLE 75G)	26	9

Food	Measure	✗ Risk-Points	✓ Life-Points
WHEAT GERM	toasted plain (1 CUP 113G)	30	50
	toasted with brown sugar and honey (1 CUP 113G)	22	42
WHEATENA	cooked with water (wheat) (¾ CUP 182G)	2	4
WHOLE WHEAT	hot natural cereal cooked with water (¾ CUP 182G)	1	5

Breads

Food	Measure	✗ Risk-Points	✓ Life-Points
BAGELS	cinnamon-raisin, toasted (3½" BAGEL 66G)	2	7
	egg, toasted (3½" BAGEL 66G)	3	8
	oat bran, toasted (3½" BAGEL 66G)	2	8
	plain toasted (includes onion, poppy, and sesame) (3½" BAGEL 66G)	2	4
BANANA BREAD	prepared from recipe (1 SLICE 60G)	15	4
BOSTON BROWN BREAD	canned (1 SLICE 45G)	1	2
BREAD CRUMBS	grated (1 CUP 120G)	7	12
BREAD STICKS	plain (1 STICK 10G)	2	1
CORNBREAD	prepared from dry mix (1 PIECE 60G)	15	5

Food	Measure	X Risk-Points	✓ Life-Points
	made with lowfat (2%) milk (1 PIECE 60G)	10	7
	made with whole milk (1 PIECE 65G)	12	8
CRACKED-WHEAT BREAD	(1 SLICE 25G)	2	3
CROISSANTS	apple (1 CROISSANT 57G)	18	4
	butter (1 CROISSANT 57G)	50	6
	cheese (1 CROISSANT 57G)	41	8
	chocolate (1 CROISSANT 57G)	68	7
	one croissant with egg and cheese (127G)	105	16
	one croissant with egg, cheese, and bacon (129G)	115	17
	one croissant with egg, cheese, and ham (152G)	131	21
	one croissant with egg, cheese, and sausage (160G)	136	24
EGG BREAD	(1 SLICE 40G)	6	6
FRENCH OR VIENNA BREAD, INCLUDES SOURDOUGH	(1 MED SLICE 25G)	1	3
FRENCH TOAST	frozen ready-to-heat (1 PIECE 59G)	8	11
	made with lowfat (2%) milk (1 SLICE 65G)	17	6

Food	Measure	✗ Risk-Points	✓ Life-Points
	stick (28G)	14	3
	two slices with butter (135G)	58	16
IRISH SODA BREAD	(1 SLICE 60G)	7	5
ITALIAN BREAD	(1 SLICE 30G)	2	4
MIXED-GRAIN BREAD	includes whole-grain, 7-grain (1 SLICE 26G)	2	4
MUFFINS	blueberry made with lowfat (2%) milk (1 MUFFIN 57G)	15	6
	blueberry made with whole milk (1 MUFFIN 57G)	16	5
	blueberry toaster-type (1 TOASTED MUFFIN 31G)	7	1
	corn made with lowfat (2%) milk (1 MUFFIN 57G)	17	7
	corn made with whole milk (1 MUFFIN 57G)	18	7
	corn toaster-type (1 TOASTED MUFFIN 31G)	9	2
	English mixed-grain, toasted (includes granola) (1 MUFFIN 61G)	2	8
	English raisin-cinnamon toasted (includes apple-cinnamon) (1 MUFFIN 52G)	3	6
	English wheat toasted (1 MUFFIN 52G)	2	7

Food	Measure	✗ Risk-Points	✓ Life-Points
	English whole wheat toasted (1 MUFFIN 61G)	3	8
	English with butter (1 MUFFIN 63G)	18	9
	English with cheese and sausage (1 MUFFIN 115G)	73	19
	English with egg, cheese, and Canadian bacon (1 MUFFIN 146G)	67	22
	English with egg, cheese, and sausage (1 MUFFIN 165G)	93	29
	oat bran (1 MUFFIN 57G)	10	6
	plain made with lowfat (2%) milk (1 MUFFIN 57G)	16	6
	plain made with whole milk (1 MUFFIN 57G)	17	6
	wheat bran made with lowfat (2%) milk (1 MUFFIN 57G)	17	10
	wheat bran made with whole milk (1 MUFFIN 57G)	18	10
	wheat bran toaster-type with raisins (1 TOASTED MUFFIN 34G)	7	2
OAT BRAN BREAD	regular (1 SLICE 30G)	3	4
	reduced-calorie (1 SLICE 23G)	1	2
OATMEAL BREAD	regular (1 SLICE 27G)	2	3
	reduced-calorie (1 SLICE 23G)	2	2

Food	Measure	✗ Risk-Points	✓ Life-Points
PITA BREAD	white (1 PITA 60G)	1	8
	whole wheat (1 PITA 64G)	4	8
PIZZA	with cheese (1 SLICE 63G)	11	11
	with cheese, meat, and vegetables (1 SLICE 79G)	13	11
	with pepperoni (1 SLICE 71G)	17	10
PROTEIN BREAD	(includes gluten) (1 SLICE 19G)	1	2
PUMPERNICKEL BREAD	(1 SLICE 32G)	2	4
PUMPKIN BREAD	(1 SLICE 60G)	19	4
RAISIN BREAD	(1 SLICE 26G)	2	3
	unenriched (1 SLICE 26G)	2	2
ROLLS	dinner egg (1 ROLL 35G)	5	6
	dinner plain commercially prepared (includes brown-and-serve) (1 AVERAGE 66G)	12	9
	dinner plain made with lowfat (2%) milk (1 ROLL 35G)	6	4
	dinner plain made with whole milk (1 ROLL 35G)	6	4
	dinner rye (1 ROLL 28G)	2	3
	dinner wheat (1 ROLL 28G)	4	3
	french (1 ROLL 38G)	4	5

Food	Measure	✗ Risk-Points	✓ Life-Points
	hamburger or hot dog, mixed-grain (1 ROLL 43G)	6	6
	hamburger or hot dog, plain (1 ROLL 43G)	5	5
	hamburger or hot dog, reduced-calorie (1 ROLL 43G)	2	6
	hard (includes kaiser) (1 ROLL 57G)	6	7
RYE BREAD	regular (1 SLICE 32G)	2	4
	reduced-calorie (1 SLICE 23G)	1	2
STUFFING	bread, plain (½ CUP 116G)	20	7
	cornbread, dry mix prepared (½ CUP 100G)	22	4
SWEET ROLLS	cheese (1 ROLL 66G)	30	5
	cinnamon, with raisins (1 ROLL 60G)	24	6
	with raisins and nuts (1 ROLL 57G)	18	6
WHEAT BREAD	includes wheat berry (1 SLICE 25G)	2	3
	reduced-calorie (1 SLICE 23G)	1	3
WHITE BREAD	commercially prepared (includes soft bread crumbs) (1 SLICE 25G)	2	3
	made with lowfat (2%) milk (1 SLICE 42G)	5	5
	made with nonfat dry milk (1 SLICE 44G)	2	5
	made with whole milk (1 SLICE 38G)	5	5

Food	Measure	✗ Risk-Points	✓ Life-Points
	reduced-calorie (1 SLICE 23G)	1	3
WHOLE WHEAT BREAD	(1 SLICE 25G)	2	3

Crackers

Food	Measure	✗ Risk-Points	✓ Life-Points
CORN CAKES	very low sodium (2 CAKES 18G)	1	1
CRACKERS	cheese, regular (10 x 1 IN SQ CRACKERS 10G)	7	2
	cheese, sandwich-type with peanut butter filling (1 SANDWICH CRACKER 7G)	4	1
	cream (1 CRACKER 7G)	2	0
	crispbread, rye (1 WAFER 10G)	0	1
	matzo, egg (1 MATZO 1 OZ 28G)	1	5
	matzo, egg and onion (1 MATZO 1 OZ 28G)	2	4
	matzo, plain (1 MATZO 1 OZ 28G)	0	3
	matzo, whole-wheat (1 MATZO 1 OZ 28G)	1	5
	melba toast, plain (1 TOAST 5G)	0	0
	melba toast, rye (includes pumpernickel) (1 TOAST 5G)	0	0

Food	Measure	X Risk-Points	✓ Life-Points
	melba toast, wheat (1 TOAST 5G)	0	0
	milk (1 CRACKER 12G)	4	1
	rusk toast (1 RUSK 10G)	1	1
	rye wafers, plain (1 TRIPLE CRACKER 25G)	0	3
	rye wafers, seasoned (1 TRIPLE CRACKER 22G)	5	2
	saltines (includes oyster, soda, soup) (3 CRACKERS 9G)	2	1
	standard snack-type, regular (3 ROUND CRACKERS 9G)	5	1
	standard snack-type, sandwich with peanut butter filling (1 SANDWICH CRACKER 7G)	4	1
	wheat (3 CRACKERS 6G)	3	0
	wheat, sandwich with cheese filling (1 SANDWICH CRACKER 7G)	4	1
	wheat, sandwich with peanut butter filling (1 SANDWICH CRACKER 7G)	4	1
	whole wheat (3 SQ CRACKERS 12G)	5	1
CRISPBREAD	rye (1 PIECE 6G)	0	0
OATCAKES	(1 BISCUIT 10G)	4	1
PRETZELS	(10 TWISTS 60G)	5	8

Food	Measure	✗ Risk-Points	✓ Life-Points
RICE CAKES	brown rice and buckwheat (2 CAKES 18G)	1	2
	brown rice and corn (2 CAKES 18G)	1	1
	brown rice, multigrain (2 CAKES 18G)	1	2
	brown rice, plain (2 CAKES 18G)	1	2
	brown rice and rye (2 CAKES 18G)	1	1
	brown rice and sesame seed (2 CAKES 18G)	1	2
WATER BISCUITS	(3 BISCUITS 15G)	4	1
ZWIEBACK	(1 PIECE 7G)	2	0

Grains

Food	Measure	✗ Risk-Points	✓ Life-Points
AMARANTH	boiled (½ CUP 66G)	0	6
BARLEY	pearl, cooked (½ CUP 79G)	0	4
BUCKWHEAT	groats, roasted (½ CUP 99G)	1	3
BULGUR	cooked (½ CUP 91G)	0	4
CORN	cooked (½ CUP 70G)	1	2
COUSCOUS	cooked (½ CUP 90G)	0	3
HOMINY	canned, white (½ CUP 80G)	1	1

Food	Measure	Risk-Points ✗	Life-Points ✓
MILLET	cooked (½ CUP 120G)	3	6
OAT BRAN	cooked (½ CUP 110G)	2	3
OATS	regular, quick, and instant, cooked with water (½ CUP 117G)	2	3
QUINOA	(½ CUP 85G)	12	16
RICE	brown, long-grain, cooked (½ CUP 98G)	2	3
	brown, medium-grain, cooked (½ CUP 98G)	2	3
	white, glutinous, cooked (½ CUP 120G)	0	1
	white, long-grain parboiled, enriched (½ CUP 88G)	0	3
	white, long-grain precooked or instant, enriched, cooked (½ CUP 82G)	0	2
	white, long-grain regular, cooked (½ CUP 79G)	0	3
	white, medium-grain, cooked (½ CUP 93G)	0	3
	white, short-grain, cooked (½ CUP 93G)	0	3
	white, with pasta, cooked (½ CUP 101G)	7	5
WHEAT GERM	crude (½ CUP 58G)	14	32
	crude (2 TBSP 14G)	3	8

Food	Measure	✗ Risk-Points	✓ Life-Points
WHEAT	sprouted (½ CUP 54G)	1	5
WILD RICE	cooked (½ CUP 82G)	0	4

Pasta

Food	Measure	✗ Risk-Points	✓ Life-Points
CANNELLONI	cheesy vegetable filling (3 SHELLS 300G)	76	10
	meat-filled (3 SHELLS 300G)	42	24
	spinach and ricotta (3 SHELLS 300G)	56	12
LASAGNE	made with ground beef and Parmesan (1 SERVING 300G)	75	34
	vegetarian, made with textured vegetable protein and Parmesan (1 SERVING 300G)	25	44
MACARONI	cheese (1 SERVING 200G)	74	12
	cheese, canned (1 SERVING 205G)	35	11
	cooked, enriched (1 CUP 140G)	2	7
	protein-fortified, cooked, enriched (1 CUP 115G)	0	7
	vegetable, cooked, enriched (1 CUP 134G)	0	5
	whole-wheat, cooked (1 CUP 140G)	1	6
NOODLES	Chinese chow mein (1 CUP 45G)	34	7

Food	Measure	✗ Risk-Points	✓ Life-Points
	egg, cooked, enriched (1 CUP 160G)	5	9
	egg, spinach, cooked, enriched (1 CUP 160G)	6	12
	Japanese soba, cooked (1 CUP 114G)	0	3
	Japanese somen, cooked (1 CUP 176G)	0	2
PASTA	e fagoli soup, homemade (1 CUP 253G)	12	10
	fresh-refrigerated, plain, cooked (1 CUP 140G)	3	8
	fresh-refrigerated, spinach, cooked (1 CUP 140G)	3	9
	homemade, made with egg, cooked (1 CUP 140G)	6	8
	homemade, made without egg, cooked (1 CUP 140G)	3	7
	salad (pasta, vegetables, and mayonnaise) (1 SERVING 180G)	33	7
	salad, wholemeal (pasta, vegetables, and mayonnaise) (1 SERVING 180G)	33	10
PASTITSIO	(Greek macaroni, lentils, and vegetables with white sauce) (1 SERVING 180G)	48	12
SPAGHETTI	bolognese, with meat sauce (1 SERVING 410G)	57	32
	cooked, enriched (1 CUP 140G)	2	7

Food	Measure	X Risk-Points	✓ Life-Points
	in four-cheese sauce (Gruyère, fontina, Parmesan, and mozzarella) (1 SERVING 449G)	317	42
	protein-fortified, cooked enriched (1 CUP 140G)	0	10
	whole wheat, cooked (1 CUP 140G)	1	6
	with Italian sauce (tomatoes, mushrooms, ham, olive oil) (1 SERVING 382G)	49	18
	with pesto sauce (1 SERVING 255G)	43	16
	with simple tomato sauce (made from tomatoes, onion, garlic, olive oil, and green pepper) (1 SERVING 300G)	26	11
TAGLIATELLE	with vegetables (1 SERVING 300G)	22	5

LifePoints Food Group Three: Vegetables and Vegetable Products

General

Food	Measure	X Risk-Points	✓ Life-Points
ALFALFA	seeds, sprouted, raw (1 CUP 33G)	0	2
AMARANTH	boiled (1 CUP 132G)	0	13
ARTICHOKES	globe or French, boiled, drained (½ CUP HEARTS 84G)	0	6

Food	Measure	✗ Risk-Points	✓ Life-Points
ARUGULA	raw (½ CUP 10G)	0	1
ASPARAGUS	boiled (4 SPEARS ½" BASE 60G)	0	7
	canned (½ CUP SPEARS 121G)	1	11
	raw (4 SPEARS 58G)	0	6
	soup, cream of, canned condensed (1 CUP 251G)	20	9
	soup, cream of, canned prep with eq vol milk (1 CUP 248G)	24	10
	soup, cream of, canned prep with eq vol water (1 CUP 244G)	10	4
	soup, cream of, dehydrated prep with water (1 CUP 251G)	4	2
BAMBOO SHOOTS	boiled (1 CUP ½" SLICES 120G)	0	2
	canned (1 CUP ⅛" SLICES 131G)	1	3
BEET GREENS	boiled drained (½ CUP 1" PIECES 72G)	0	6
BEETS	boiled (½ CUP SLICES 85G)	0	5
	canned (½ CUP SLICES 123G)	0	3
	harvard, canned (½ CUP SLICES 123G)	0	3
	pickled, canned (½ CUP SLICES 114G)	0	3
BROCCOLI	boiled (1 SPEAR 180G)	1	13
	boiled (½ CUP CHOPPED 78G)	0	5
	flower clusters, raw (1 CLUSTER 151G)	1	14

Food	Measure	✗ Risk-Points	✓ Life-Points
	flower clusters, raw (½ CUP CHOPPED 44G)	0	4
	frozen, chopped, boiled (½ CUP 92G)	0	6
	raw (1 SPEAR 151G)	1	14
	stalks, raw (1 SPEAR 151G)	1	13
BRUSSEL SPROUTS	boiled (½ CUP 78G)	0	6
	frozen, boiled (½ CUP 78G)	0	8
	raw (5 SPROUTS 55G)	0	5
BURDOCK ROOT	boiled (1 CUP 1″ PIECES 125G)	0	6
	raw (1 CUP 1″ PIECES 118G)	0	5
CABBAGE, CHINESE (BOK CHOY)	boiled drained with salt (½ CUP SHREDDED 85G)	0	5
	boiled drained without salt (½ CUP SHREDDED 85G)	0	5
	raw (½ CUP SHREDDED 35G)	0	2
CABBAGE, CHINESE (PO-TSAI)	boiled (½ CUP SHREDDED 60G)	0	3
	raw (½ CUP SHREDDED 38G)	0	3
CABBAGE, COMMON	Danish, domestic, red, and pointed types, boiled (½ CUP SHREDDED 75G)	0	2
	raw (½ CUP SHREDDED 35G)	0	1

Food	Measure	Risk-Points	Life-Points
	savoy, boiled (1/2 CUP SHREDDED 73G)	0	3
	savoy, raw (1/2 CUP SHREDDED 35G)	0	2
CARDOON	boiled (1 AVERAGE 4 OZ SERVING 115G)	0	3
	raw (1/2 CUP 89G)	0	3
CARROT JUICE	canned (1/2 CUP 123G)	0	11
CARROTS	boiled (1/2 CUP SLICES 78G)	0	7
	canned (1/2 CUP SLICES 73G)	0	4
	frozen, boiled (1/2 CUP SLICES 73G)	0	4
	raw (1/2 CUP SHREDDED 55G)	0	5
	raw (1 CARROT 7 1/2" 72G)	0	7
CAULIFLOWER	boiled (1/2 CUP 1" PIECES 62G)	0	3
	frozen, boiled (1/2 CUP 1" PIECES 90G)	0	3
	raw (1/2 CUP 1" PIECES 50G)	0	3
	soup, dehydrated prep with water (1 CUP 256G)	4	3
CELERIAC (CELERY ROOT)	boiled drained (1 CUP DICED 150G)	0	3
	raw (1/2 CUP 78G)	0	3
CELERY	boiled drained (1/2 CUP DICED 75G)	0	2
	raw (1 STALK 40G)	0	1
	raw (1/2 CUP DICED 60G)	0	2

Food	Measure	✗ Risk-Points	✓ Life-Points
	soup, cream of, canned prep with eq vol milk (1 CUP 248G)	29	8
	soup, cream of, canned prep with eq vol water (1 CUP 244G)	13	3
	soup, cream of, dehydrated prep with water (1 CUP 254G)	4	2
CHARD, SWISS	boiled drained (½ CUP CHOPPED 88G)	0	4
	raw (½ CUP CHOPPED 18G)	0	0
CHAYOTE	boiled drained (½ CUP 1" PIECES 80G)	0	2
CHICORY	greens, raw (½ CUP CHOPPED 90G)	0	10
	roots, raw (½ CUP 1" PIECES 45G)	0	1
CHIVES	freeze-dried (¼ CUP 1G)	0	0
	raw (1 TBSP CHOPPED 3G)	0	0
COLLARDS	boiled drained (½ CUP CHOPPED 64G)	0	1
	frozen, chopped, boiled (½ CUP CHOPPED 85G)	0	9
CORN ON THE COB	with butter (1 EAR 146G)	12	9
CORN	sweet white, boiled (½ CUP CUT 82G)	2	5
	sweet white, canned (½ CUP 82G)	2	4
	sweet white, canned, cream style (½ CUP 128G)	1	5

Food	Measure	✗ Risk-Points	✓ Life-Points
	sweet white, frozen kernels, boiled (½ CUP 82G)	0	3
	sweet white, raw (½ CUP CUT 77G)	2	5
	sweet yellow, boiled drained (½ CUP CUT 82G)	2	5
	sweet yellow, canned (½ CUP 82G)	2	4
	sweet yellow, canned, cream style (½ CUP 128G)	1	6
	sweet yellow, frozen kernels, boiled (½ CUP 82G)	0	3
	sweet yellow, raw (½ CUP CUT 77G)	2	5
CORN SALAD (MÂCHE)	raw (½ CUP 28G)	0	2
CRESS, GARDEN	boiled drained (½ CUP 68G)	1	5
	raw (½ CUP 25G)	0	3
CUCUMBER	raw (½ CUP SLICES 52G)	0	1
DANDELION GREENS	boiled (½ CUP CHOPPED 52G)	0	5
	raw (½ CUP CHOPPED 28G)	0	3
EGGPLANT	sautéed in olive oil (½ CUP CUBES 64G)	35	1
	boiled (½ CUP 1" CUBES 48G)	0	1
ENDIVE	raw (½ CUP CHOPPED 25G)	0	2
	Belgian endive, raw (½ CUP 45G)	0	1

Food	Measure	✗ Risk-Points	✓ Life-Points
ESCAROLE	soup, canned ready-to-serve (1 CUP 248G)	4	9
FENNEL	bulb raw (1 CUP SLICED 87G)	0	3
GARLIC	raw (3 CLOVES 9G)	0	1
GAZPACHO	canned ready-to-serve (1 CUP 244G)	5	5
GINGER	root raw (¼ CUP 1″ DIAM SLICES 24G)	0	0
JERUSALEM ARTICHOKE	boiled (½ CUP SLICES 75G)	0	1
KALE	boiled (½ CUP CHOPPED 65G)	0	4
KOHLRABI	boiled (½ CUP SLICES 82G)	0	2
	raw (½ CUP SLICES 70G)	0	3
LEEKS	bulb and lower leaf portion boiled (1 LEEK 124G)	0	4
	soup, dehydrated prep with water (1 CUP 254G)	0	4
LETTUCE	butterhead (includes Boston and Bibb types) raw (1 HEAD 5″ DIAM 163G)	0	10
	cos or romaine raw (½ CUP SHREDDED 28G)	0	3
	iceberg (includes crisphead types) raw (1 LEAF 20G)	0	0
	looseleaf raw (½ CUP SHREDDED 28G)	0	1
LOTUS ROOT	boiled drained (10 SLCS 2½″ DIAM 89G)	0	3

Food	Measure	✗ Risk-Points	✓ Life-Points
MINESTRONE SOUP	canned prep with eq vol water (1 CUP 241G)	6	5
	canned chunky ready-to-serve (1 CUP 240G)	11	9
	dehydrated prep with water (1 CUP 254G)	6	4
MUSHROOM	sautéed in corn oil (1 MUSHROOM 21G)	8	1
	raw (1 MUSHROOM 18G)	0	1
	raw (½ CUP PIECES 35G)	0	3
	shiitake, dried (4 MUSHROOMS 15G)	0	5
	shiitake, sautéed in corn oil (4 MUSHROOMS 20G)	8	5
MUSHROOM SOUP	cream of, canned prep with eq vol milk (1 CUP 248G)	38	8
	cream of, canned prep with eq vol water (1 CUP 244G)	22	3
	dehydrated prep with water (1 CUP 253G)	12	5
	with beef stock canned prep with eq vol water (1 CUP 244G)	11	4
	with barley, canned prep with eq vol water (1 CUP 244G)	5	3
MUSTARD GREENS	boiled (½ CUP CHOPPED 70G)	0	5
	raw (1 CUP CHOPPED 56G)	0	9

Food	Measure	X Risk-Points	✓ Life-Points
OKRA	sautéed in corn oil (½ CUP SLICES 92G)	60	12
ONION	boiled drained (½ CUP CHOPPED 105G)	0	3
	canned (½ CUP CHOPPED 112G)	0	2
	dehydrated flakes (¼ CUP 14G)	0	4
	raw (½ CUP CHOPPED 80G)	0	2
	rings, breaded and fried (3 RINGS 30G)	18	1
	sautéed in olive oil (¼ CUP 60G)	13	1
	soup canned prep with eq vol water (1 CUP 241G)	4	3
	soup, cream of, canned prep with eq vol milk (1 CUP 248G)	30	9
	soup, cream of, canned prep with eq vol water (1 CUP 244G)	13	2
	soup, dehydrated prep with water (1 CUP 246G)	1	1
	spring (scallions) raw (½ CUP CHOPPED 50G)	0	3
PARSLEY	raw (½ CUP CHOPPED 30G)	0	5
PARSNIPS	boiled (½ CUP SLICES 78G)	0	5
PEPPERS	hot chile, green, raw (½ CUP CHOPPED 75G)	0	6
	hot chile, red, raw (½ CUP CHOPPED 75G)	0	8

Food	Measure	Risk-Points	Life-Points
	jalapeño, canned (½ CUP CHOPPED 68G)	1	3
	sweet green canned (½ CUP HALVES 70G)	0	2
	sweet green raw (1 PEPPER 74G)	0	3
	sweet green, sautéed (½ CUP CHOPPED 68G)	12	3
	sweet red, canned (½ CUP HALVES 70G)	0	1
	sweet red raw (1 PEPPER 74G)	0	5
	sweet red, sautéed (½ CUP CHOPPED 68G)	12	4
	sweet yellow, raw (1 PEPPER 74G)	0	4
PIMIENTO	canned (1 TBSP 12G)	0	0
POI	(½ CUP 120G)	0	6
PUMPKIN	boiled drained (½ CUP MASHED 122G)	0	3
	canned (½ CUP 122G)	1	7
	pie mix, canned (½ CUP 135G)	0	9
PURSLANE	boiled (½ CUP 58G)	0	2
	raw (½ CUP 22G)	0	1
RADICCHIO	raw (½ CUP SHREDDED 20G)	0	0
RADISH	seeds sprouted raw (½ CUP 19G)	1	2
	oriental boiled (½ CUP SLICES 74G)	0	1

Food	Measure	✗ Risk-Points	✓ Life-Points
	oriental raw (½ CUP SLICES 44G)	0	1
	raw (½ CUP SLICES 58G)	0	1
	raw (10 RADISHES ¾"–1" 45G)	0	1
	white icicle raw (½ CUP SLICES 50G)	0	1
RATATOUILLE	(½ CUP 107G)	30	3
RUTABAGA	boiled (½ CUP CUBES 85G)	0	3
SALAD, MIXED	without dressing—add dressing from food group 6 (1 AVERAGE SERVING 115G)	0	5
	without dressing, with cheese and egg (1 AVERAGE SERVING 115G)	11	6
	without dressing, with pasta and seafood (1 AVERAGE SERVING 115G)	14	7
	without dressing, with shrimp (1 AVERAGE SERVING 115G)	3	12
	without dressing, with turkey, ham, and cheese (1 AVERAGE SERVING 115G)	21	10
SALSIFY (OYSTER PLANT)	boiled (½ CUP SLICES 68G)	0	3
SAUERKRAUT	canned (½ CUP 118G)	0	4
SEAWEED	kelp raw (STANDARD 1 OZ SERVING 28G)	0	4
	laver raw (STANDARD 1 OZ SERVING 28G)	0	4

Food	Measure	Risk-Points ✗	Life-Points ✓
	spirulina dried (STANDARD 1 OZ SERVING 28G)	5	22
	wakame raw (STANDARD 1 OZ SERVING 28G)	0	4
SHALLOTS	raw (1 TBSP CHOPPED 10G)	0	0
SPINACH	boiled (½ CUP 90G)	0	15
	canned (½ CUP 107G)	1	12
	frozen, cooked (½ CUP 95G)	0	12
	soufflé (1 AVERAGE SERVING 115G)	45	15
SQUASH	summer, all varieties inc zucchini, boiled (½ CUP SLICES 90G)	0	2
	winter, all varieties, baked (½ CUP CUBES 102G)	1	5
STOCKPOT SOUP	canned prep with eq vol water (1 CUP 247G)	9	5
SUCCOTASH (CORN AND LIMAS)	boiled (1 CUP 96G)	1	6
	canned with corn (½ CUP 133G)	1	6
	frozen, boiled (½ CUP 85G)	1	5
SWEET POTATO	baked in skin (½ CUP MASHED 100G)	0	10
	candied (1 PIECE 2½" x 2" 105G)	10	3
	canned (½ CUP 127G)	0	9
TOMATILLOS	raw (½ CUP CHOPPED 66G)	1	2

Food	Measure	✗ Risk-Points	✓ Life-Points
TOMATO	bisque canned prep with eq vol milk (1 CUP 251G)	23	10
	bisque canned prep with eq vol water (1 CUP 247G)	6	4
	green, raw (1 TOMATO 2⅗" 123G)	0	3
	juice, canned (½ CUP 122G)	0	4
	paste, canned (1 TBSP 16G)	0	1
	paste, canned (½ CUP 131G)	2	15
	purée, canned (½ CUP 125G)	0	6
	ripe red, stewed (½ CUP 51G)	3	2
	ripe red, canned (½ CUP 131G)	0	3
	sauce, canned (½ CUP 122G)	0	5
	soup, canned prep with eq vol milk (1 CUP 248G)	21	11
	soup, canned prep with eq vol water (1 CUP 244G)	4	5
	soup, dehydrated prep with water (1 CUP 265G)	8	3
	soup and rice, canned prep with eq vol water (1 CUP 247G)	6	4
	soup and vegetable, dehydrated prep with water (1 CUP 253G)	2	2
	sun-dried (½ CUP 27G)	2	7
	sun-dried packed in oil, drained (½ CUP 27G)	9	3

Food	Measure	✗ Risk-Points	✓ Life-Points
TURNIP GREENS	boiled (½ CUP CHOPPED 72G)	0	8
TURNIPS	boiled (½ CUP CUBES 78G)	0	1
	raw (½ CUP CUBES 65G)	0	2
VEGETABLE JUICE	cocktail (½ CUP 121G)	0	4
VEGETABLE SOUP	canned chunky ready-to-serve (1 CUP 240G)	9	8
	dehydrated cream of, prep with water (1 CUP 260G)	14	10
	vegetarian, canned prep with eq vol water (1 CUP 241G)	4	4
	canned with beef broth, prep with eq vol water (1 CUP 241G)	4	4
VEGETABLES, MIXED	canned (½ CUP 82G)	0	5
	frozen, boiled (½ CUP 91G)	0	4
WATER CHESTNUTS	Chinese, canned (½ CUP SLICES 70G)	0	1
WATERCRESS	raw (½ CUP CHOPPED 17G)	0	1
YAM	boiled or baked (½ CUP CUBES 68G)	0	3

Potato Products

Food	Measure	✗ Risk-Points	✓ Life-Points
AU GRATIN	dry mix prepared with water, whole milk, and butter (⅙ OF 5.5-OZ PK 137G)	26	4
	prepared using butter (½ CUP 122G)	43	7
	prepared using margarine (½ CUP 122G)	32	7
BAKED	topped with cheese sauce (1 POTATO 296G)	79	18
	topped with cheese sauce and bacon (1 POTATO 299G)	15	21
	topped with cheese sauce and broccoli (1 POTATO 339G)	63	23
	topped with cheese sauce and chile (1 POTATO 395G)	97	28
	topped with sour cream and chives (1 POTATO 302G)	75	16
	flesh and skin (FROM 2⅓" x 4¾" POTATO 202G)	0	12
BOILED	flesh only (½ CUP 61G)	0	2
	skin only (SKIN FROM 1 POTATO 58G)	0	7
	in skin (½ CUP 78G)	0	3
	flesh only (½ CUP 78G)	0	3

Food	Measure	✗ Risk-Points	✓ Life-Points
CANNED	(½ CUP 150G)	0	5
CURRY	potato and cauliflower pakora/bhajia, fried in vegetable oil (1 AVERAGE SERVING 115G)	63	11
	potato and green pepper bhaji (1 AVERAGE SERVING 115G)	26	5
	potato and pea curry (1 AVERAGE SERVING 115G)	10	6
	potato bhaji, with butter ghee (1 AVERAGE SERVING 115G)	55	6
	potato, carrot, and pea pakora/bhajia, fried in vegetable oil (1 AVERAGE SERVING 115G)	64	15
	potato, onion, and mushroom bhaji (1 AVERAGE SERVING 115G)	50	6
	potato pakora/bhajia, fried in vegetable oil (1 AVERAGE SERVING 115G)	56	13
FLOUR	(½ CUP 90G)	1	18
FRENCH FRIED	from fresh, fried in beef tallow and veg oil (AVERAGE SERVING 76G)	37	5
	from fresh, fried in beef tallow (AVERAGE SERVING 76G)	42	5
	from fresh, fried in vegetable oil (AVERAGE SERVING 76G)	30	5
	from frozen, par-fried cottage-cut prepared htd/oven (10 STRIPS 50G)	14	3

Food	Measure	✗ Risk-Points	✓ Life-Points
	from frozen, par-fried prepared htd/oven (10 STRIPS 50G)	28	3
	from frozen, par-fried restaurant-prepared fried in animal fat and veg oil (10 STRIPS 50G)	25	3
	from frozen, par-fried restaurant-prepared fried in veg oil (10 STRIPS 50G)	20	3
HASHED BROWN	(½ CUP 72G)	32	3
	prepared from frozen, plain (½ CUP 78G)	26	3
MASHED	dehydrated—prepared with whole milk and butter (½ CUP 105G)	27	3
	dehydrated—prepared with water and margarine (½ CUP 105G)	5	3
	homemade, whole milk added (½ CUP 105G)	2	4
	homemade, whole milk and butter added (½ CUP 105G)	21	4
	home-prepared, whole milk and margarine added (½ CUP 105G)	11	4
MICROWAVED	cooked in skin, flesh and skin eaten (POTATO 2⅓" x 4¾" 202G)	0	11
	cooked in skin, flesh only eaten (½ CUP 78G)	0	3
	cooked in skin, skin only eaten (SKIN FROM 1 POTATO 58G)	0	5

Food	Measure	X Risk-Points	✓ Life-Points
POTATO O'BRIEN	prepared from frozen (1 4 OZ SERVING 115G)	37	6
	homemade (1 CUP 194G)	11	8
POTATO PANCAKES	homemade (1 PANCAKE 76G)	28	7
POTATO PUFFS	prepared from frozen (½ CUP 62G)	23	4
POTATO SALAD	with mayonnaise (½ CUP 125G)	82	5
	with reduced calorie dressing (½ CUP 125G)	12	4
SCALLOPED POTATO	dry mix prepared with water, whole milk, and butter (⅙ of 5.5 OZ PK 137G)	27	4
	homemade with butter (½ CUP 122G)	20	5
	homemade with margarine (½ CUP 122G)	12	5
SOUP	cream of potato, canned prepared with eq vol milk (1 CUP 248G)	28	8
	cream of potato, canned prepared with eq vol water (1 CUP 244G)	9	2

LifePoints Food Group Four: Legumes, Nuts, and Seeds

Legumes and Beans

Food	Measure	✗ Risk-Points	✓ Life-Points
ADZUKI BEANS	boiled (½ CUP 115G)	0	13
BAKED BEANS	canned with franks (½ CUP 128G)	22	9
	canned with pork (½ CUP 126G)	5	8
	canned with pork plus sweet sauce (½ CUP 126G)	5	9
	canned with pork plus tomato sauce (½ CUP 126G)	3	12
	canned, plain or vegetarian (½ CUP 127G)	1	8
	homemade (½ CUP 126G)	18	10
BARBECUE BEANS	canned in sauce (½ CUP 126G)	1	4
BEAN AND LENTIL CHILI	(½ CUP 126G)	8	8
BEAN AND MIXED VEGETABLE CASSEROLE	(½ CUP 126G)	2	7
BEAN SALAD	purchased (½ CUP 126G)	29	8
BEAN SOUP	dehydrated with bacon, prep with water (1 CUP 265G)	7	6

Food	Measure	Risk-Points	Life-Points
	canned with frankfurters, prep with eq vol water (1 CUP 250G)	17	8
	chunky canned with ham, ready-to-serve (1 CUP 243G)	24	13
	canned with pork, prep with eq vol water (1 CUP 253G)	14	8
BLACK BEANS	boiled or canned (½ CUP 86G)	1	11
	soup, canned prep with eq vol water (1 CUP 247G)	3	7
BLACK TURTLE BEANS	boiled or canned (½ CUP 120G)	0	9
BROAD BEANS (FAVA BEANS)	boiled or canned (½ 128G)	0	7
BUTTER BEANS	boiled or canned (½ CUP 80G)	1	3
CHICK-PEAS (GARBANZO BEAN)	and potato curry (½ CUP 126G)	17	7
	and tomato curry, with butter ghee (½ CUP 126G)	80	12
	and tomato curry, with vegetable oil (½ CUP 126G)	45	11
	boiled or canned (½ CUP 120G)	3	12
	falafel (2¼" PATTY 17G)	7	2
	hummus (⅓ CUP 82G)	17	8
CHILI WITH BEANS	canned (½ CUP 128G)	22	10

Food	Measure	✗ Risk-Points	✓ Life-Points
COWPEA (BLACK-EYED CROWDER SOUTHERN)	boiled (½ CUP 86G)	1	12
	canned, plain (½ CUP 120G)	1	7
	canned, with pork (½ CUP 120G)	5	7
CRANBERRY (ROMAN) BEANS	boiled (½ CUP 88G)	1	13
	canned (½ CUP 130G)	0	9
DHAL	made with mung beans (½ CUP 126G)	12	7
FRENCH BEANS	boiled (½ CUP 86G)	1	7
	raw (½ CUP 92G)	4	22
GREAT NORTHERN BEANS	boiled (½ CUP 88G)	0	9
	canned (½ CUP 131G)	1	13
GREEN PEA SOUP	canned prep with eq vol milk (1 CUP 254G)	30	12
	canned prep with eq vol water (1 CUP 250G)	10	6
	dehydrated mix prep with water (1 CUP 271G)	3	9
KIDNEY BEANS	and mung bean curry (½ CUP 126G)	38	4
	boiled (½ CUP 88G)	1	11

Food	Measure	✗ Risk-Points	✓ Life-Points
	canned (½ CUP 128G)	0	8
LENTILS	boiled (½ CUP 99G)	0	16
	curry, red/masoor dhal and tomato, with butter (½ CUP 126G)	29	4
	curry, red/masoor dhal and tomato, with vegetable oil (½ CUP 126G)	18	4
	soup, canned with ham, ready-to-serve (1 CUP 248G)	8	11
	soup, canned (1 CUP 240G)	1	7
	soup, homemade (1 CUP 240G)	54	11
	sprouted, raw (½ CUP 38G)	0	5
	sprouted, stir-fried (½ CUP 45G)	0	2
LIMA BEANS	boiled or canned (½ CUP 124G)	0	6
MULLIGATAWNY SOUP	(1 CUP 245G)	67	7
MUNG BEANS	boiled (½ CUP 101G)	0	12
	curry (½ CUP 126G)	18	7
	dhal and spinach (½ CUP 126G)	9	16
	dhal and tomato (½ CUP 126G)	11	6
	dhal, plain (½ CUP 126G)	19	4
	sprouted, boiled (½ CUP 62G)	0	2
	sprouted, canned (½ CUP 62G)	0	1

Food	Measure	✗ Risk-Points	✓ Life-Points
	sprouted, raw (½ CUP 52G)	0	3
	sprouted, stir-fried (½ CUP 62G)	0	5
NAVY BEANS	boiled or canned (½ CUP 131G)	1	12
	sprouted, boiled (½ CUP 85G)	1	12
	sprouted, raw (½ CUP 52G)	0	7
PEAS	and carrots, canned (½ CUP 128G)	0	7
	and onions, canned (½ CUP 60G)	0	3
	and potato curry (½ CUP 126G)	34	5
	bhaji (½ CUP 126G)	206	11
	green, boiled (½ CUP 80G)	0	8
	green, canned (½ CUP 85G)	0	6
	green, frozen, boiled (½ CUP 80G)	0	7
	green, raw (½ CUP 72G)	0	8
	snow peas, boiled, drained (½ CUP 80G)	0	5
	snow peas, raw (½ CUP 72G)	0	5
	split, boiled (½ CUP 98G)	0	8
PETIT POIS	canned, drained (½ CUP 85G)	1	6
	frozen, boiled (½ CUP 80G)	1	7
PINK BEANS	boiled (½ CUP 84G)	1	13
PINTO BEANS	boiled (½ CUP 85G)	1	13

Food	Measure	X Risk-Points	✓ Life-Points
SHELL BEANS	canned (½ CUP 122G)	0	4
SMALL WHITE BEANS	boiled (½ CUP 90G)	1	12
SOYBEANS	boiled (½ CUP 86G)	19	12
	kernels, roasted and toasted (½ CUP 54G)	32	14
	sprouted, steamed (½ CUP 47G)	5	4
	sprouted, stir-fried (½ CUP 47G)	8	7
SPLIT PEA SOUP	chunky canned with ham, ready-to-serve (1 CUP 240G)	11	11
	canned with ham, prep with eq vol water (1 CUP 253G)	13	7
SUGAR SNAPS	boiled (½ CUP 80G)	0	4
	raw (½ CUP 72G)	0	5
	sautéed in blended oil (½ CUP 60G)	7	4
WHITE BEANS	canned (½ CUP 131G)	0	12
	boiled (½ CUP 90G)	0	9
YELLOW BEANS	boiled (½ CUP 88G)	2	9

Legume and Bean Products

Food	Measure	✗ Risk-Points	✓ Life-Points
BACON, MEATLESS	(1 STRIP 8G)	5	3
	(½ CUP 72G)	53	18
BEAN LOAF	(1 AVERAGE SERVING 115G)	20	9
BEAN PÂTÉ	made with lentils (1 SERVING 75G)	0	11
BLACK BEAN SAUCE	(½ CUP 136G)	7	15
HUMMUS	(⅓ CUP 82G)	17	8
LENTIL AND NUT ROAST	(1 AVERAGE SERVING 115G)	34	11
	with egg (1 AVERAGE SERVING 115G)	34	12
LENTIL AND RICE ROAST	(1 AVERAGE SERVING 115G)	5	4
	with egg (1 AVERAGE SERVING 115G)	6	5
LENTIL CUTLETS	fried in vegetable oil (1 CUTLET 88G)	17	7
LENTIL ROAST	(1 AVERAGE SERVING 115G)	8	9
	with egg (1 AVERAGE SERVING 115G)	10	10
MEAT EXTENDER	(1 OZ 28G)	2	21
MISO	(1 TBSP 20G)	3	2
	(½ CUP 138G)	20	16
NATTO	(½ CUP 88G)	24	13

Food	Measure	✗ Risk-Points	✓ Life-Points
RED PEA LOAF	(West Indian—made with kidney beans) (1 SERVING 115G)	10	11
SAUSAGE, MEATLESS	(1 LINK 25G)	11	9
SOY BEANBURGER	fried in vegetable oil (1 BURGER 70G)	19	7
SOY MILK	fluid (½ CUP 120G)	5	3
SOY SAUCE	made from soy and wheat (1 TBSP 18G)	0	1
	made from soy and wheat (¼ CUP 58G)	0	3
	made from soy and wheat (shoyu) low sodium (1 TBSP 18G)	0	1
SOY MINCE	granules (½ CUP 126G)	17	36
TEMPEH	(½ CUP 83G)	15	15
	burgers made with rice, fried in vegetable oil (1 BURGER 70G)	14	5
TOFU	burger (1 BURGER 70G)	7	7
	fried (1 PIECE 13G)	6	2
	raw firm (¼ BLOCK 81G)	17	15
	raw regular (¼ BLOCK 116G)	13	11
	salted and fermented (fuyu) (1 BLOCK 11G)	2	2
	steamed (½ CUP 124G)	13	11

Food	Measure	✗ Risk-Points	✓ Life-Points
	steamed, fried (½ CUP 124G)	54	19
	spread (1 TBSP 15G)	7	0
VEGETARIAN PATÉ	soya, cereal, and vegetable (1 TBSP 15G)	5	5

Nuts and Nut Products

Food	Measure	✗ Risk-Points	✓ Life-Points
ALMONDS	butter (1 TBSP 16G)	20	3
	dried (1 OZ 28G)	37	5
	dry roasted (1 OZ 28G)	36	6
	oil roasted (1 OZ OR 24 WHL KERNELS 28G)	40	5
	paste (1 OZ 28G)	19	5
	toasted (1 OZ 28G)	36	6
BRAZIL NUTS	dried (1 OZ OR 6–8 KERNELS 28G)	47	5
CASHEWS	butter (1 TBSP 16G)	19	2
	dry roasted (1 OZ 28G)	32	5
	oil roasted (1 OZ 28G)	34	5
CHESTNUTS	European, boiled and steamed (1 OZ 28G)	0	2
	European roasted (1 OZ 28G)	1	3

Food	Measure	Risk-Points ✗	Life-Points ✓
COCONUT	cream, canned (liquid expressed from grated meat) (1 TBSP 19G)	22	0
	cream, raw (liquid expressed from grated meat) (1 TBSP 15G)	34	0
	meat, raw (½ CUP SHREDDED OR GRATED 40G)	89	2
	meat, desiccated, creamed (½ CUP 40G)	183	2
	meat, desiccated, flaked (½ CUP 40G)	84	2
	meat, desiccated, shredded (½ CUP 45G)	106	2
	meat, desiccated, toasted (½ CUP 40G)	125	2
	milk, canned (liquid expressed from grated meat and water) (½ CUP 113G)	160	4
	milk, raw (liquid expressed from grated meat and water) (½ CUP 120G)	190	4
	water (liquid from coconuts) (½ CUP 120G)	1	1
COTTONSEED	kernels roasted (1 OZ 10G)	9	3
FILBERTS OR HAZELNUTS	dried (1 OZ 28G)	44	5
	dry roasted (1 OZ 28G)	47	5

Food	Measure	✗ Risk-Points	✓ Life-Points
	oil roasted (1 OZ 28G)	45	5
GINKGO NUTS	canned (1 OZ OR 14 MED KRNLS 28G)	1	2
	dried (1 OZ 28G)	1	6
	raw (1 OZ 28G)	1	3
HICKORY NUTS	dried (1 OZ 28G)	45	5
LOTUS SEEDS	dried (1 OZ OR 42 MED SEEDS 28G)	1	5
	raw (1 OZ 28G)	0	1
MACADAMIA NUTS	dried (1 OZ 28G)	52	3
	oil roasted (1 OZ OR 10–12 KERNELS 28G)	54	2
MIXED NUTS	with peanuts, dry roasted (1 OZ 28G)	36	5
	with peanuts, oil roasted (1 OZ 28G)	39	6
	without peanuts, oil roasted (1 OZ 28G)	39	5
NUT CROQUETTES	fried in vegetable oil (1 AVERAGE SERVING 115G)	75	11
NUT CUTLETS	fried in vegetable oil (1 CUTLET 88G)	49	5
	grilled (1 CUTLET 88G)	28	5
NUT ROAST	(1 AVERAGE SERVING 115G)	73	15
	with egg (1 AVERAGE SERVING 115G)	71	16
PEANUTS	boiled (½ CUP 32G)	17	4

Food	Measure	Risk-Points ✗	Life-Points ✓
	butter and banana sandwich (1 SANDWICH 201G)	51	21
	butter and jam sandwich (1 SANDWICH 127G)	50	15
	butter (1 TBSP 16G)	19	3
	dry roasted (1 OZ 28G)	34	7
	oil roasted (1 OZ 28G)	34	8
	raw (1 OZ 28G)	34	10
PECANS	dried (1 OZ 28G)	48	4
	dry roasted (1 OZ 28G)	45	3
	oil roasted (1 OZ OR 15 HALVES 28G)	50	3
PINE NUTS	pignolia dried (1 OZ OR 15 KERNELS 28G)	35	6
	pinyon dried (1 OZ 28G)	43	6
PISTACHIO NUTS	dried (1 OZ 28G)	34	6
	dry roasted (1 OZ 28G)	37	4
PUMPKIN AND SQUASH SEEDS	kernels, dried (1 OZ OR 142 KERNELS 28G)	32	7
	kernels, roasted (1 OZ 28G)	29	7
	whole, roasted (1 OZ OR 85 SEEDS 28G)	13	3
SAFFLOWER SEEDS	kernels, dried (1 OZ 28G)	27	9
SESAME SEEDS	butter paste (1 OZ 28G)	36	12

Food	Measure	Risk-Points	Life-Points
	kernels, dried (1 oz 28g)	38	8
	kernels, toasted (1 oz 28g)	34	10
	whole, dried (1 oz 28g)	34	12
	whole, roasted and toasted (1 oz 28g)	34	12
SOYBEANS	kernels, roasted and toasted (1 oz 28g)	17	7
SUNFLOWER SEEDS	butter (1 oz 28g)	33	9
	kernels, dried (1 oz 28g)	35	13
	kernels, dry roasted (1 oz 28g)	35	9
	kernels, oil roasted (1 oz 28g)	40	9
	kernels, toasted (1 oz 28g)	40	9
TAHINI	from roasted and toasted sesame kernels (1 oz 28g)	38	10
WALNUTS	black, dried (1 oz 28g)	40	4
	English or Persian dried (1 oz 28g)	43	4

LifePoints Food Group Five: Meat, Fish, and Dairy Products

Beef

Food	Measure	✗ Risk-Points	✓ Life-Points
BEEF STEW	homemade (1 CUP 252G)	13	24
BOTTOM ROUND	all grades, lean and fat, braised (3 OZ 85G)	40	20
BRISKET	lean and fat, braised (3 OZ 85G)	78	18
CHEESEBURGER	large double patty with cond and veg (1 BURGER 258G)	132	36
	large single meat patty plain (1 BURGER 185G)	111	35
	large single meat patty with bacon and cond (1 BURGER 195G)	121	32
	large single patty with cond and veg (1 BURGER 219G)	112	31
	large single patty with ham, cond, and veg (1 BURGER 254G)	158	40
	regular double patty and bun, plain (1 BURGER 160G)	71	28
	regular double patty and bun with cond and veg (1 BURGER 228G)	95	33
	regular double patty plain (1 BURGER 155G)	97	29

Food	Measure	✗ Risk-Points	✓ Life-Points
	regular double patty with cond and veg (1 BURGER 166G)	65	26
	regular single meat patty plain (1 BURGER 102G)	48	19
	regular single patty with condiments and veg (1 BURGER 154G)	68	21
	regular single patty with condiments (1 BURGER 113G)	47	16
	triple patty plain (1 BURGER 304G)	162	49
CHILI CON CARNE	(1 CUP 253G)	25	26
CHUCK ROAST	lean and fat, braised (3 OZ 85G)	65	20
CORNED BEEF	brisket (3 OZ 85G)	40	14
	canned (1 OZ 28G)	13	4
DRIED BEEF	(1 OZ 28G)	3	7
EYE OF ROUND	all grades, lean and fat, roasted (3 OZ 85G)	31	18
FLANK	lean and fat, broiled (3 OZ 85G)	33	20
GROUND	extra lean, broiled medium (3 OZ 85G)	40	19
	lean broiled, medium (3 OZ 85G)	46	19
HAMBURGER	large double patty with cond and veg (1 BURGER 226G)	78	33
	large single meat patty plain (1 BURGER 137G)	62	26

Food	Measure	Risk-Points ✗	Life-Points ✓
	large single meat patty with cond and veg (1 BURGER 218G)	78	30
	large triple patty with condiments (1 BURGER 259G)	119	42
	regular double patty plain (1 BURGER 176G)	77	31
	regular double patty with condiments (1 BURGER 215G)	90	32
	regular single patty plain (1 BURGER 90G)	31	15
	regular single patty with cond and veg (1 BURGER 110G)	33	14
	regular single patty with condiments (1 BURGER 107G)	26	16
JERKY	chopped and formed (1 LARGE PIECE 20G)	8	8
KIDNEYS	simmered (3 OZ 85G)	7	35
LIVER	braised (3 OZ 85G)	12	50
	pan-fried (3 OZ 85G)	17	53
PASTRAMI	(1 OZ 28G)	22	5
PORTERHOUSE STEAK	choice, lean and fat, broiled (3 OZ 85G)	56	19
POT ROAST	lean and fat, braised (3 OZ 85G)	59	20
RIB ROAST	all grades, lean and fat, roasted (3 OZ 85G)	74	18

Food	Measure	✗ Risk-Points	✓ Life-Points
ROUND ROAST	all grades, lean and fat, roasted (3 OZ 85G)	32	21
SANDWICH	roast beef, plain (1 SANDWICH 139G)	34	23
	roast beef, with cheese (1 SANDWICH 176G)	67	32
	steak sandwich (1 SANDWICH 204G)	35	32
	submarine with cold cuts (1 SUB 228G)	51	30
	submarine with roast beef (1 SUB 216G)	53	28
SAUSAGE	bologna, beef, and pork (1 SLICE 4½" DIAM 1 OZ 28G)	22	3
	salami, beef, and pork, cooked (1 OZ 28G)	17	7
	sausage, smoked (1 SAUSAGE 43G)	36	6
	smoked chopped beef (1 OZ 28G)	3	5
SIRLOIN	choice, lean and fat, broiled (3 OZ 85G)	39	21
	thin slices (1 OZ 28G)	3	7
SOUP	beef broth cubes prep with water (1 CUP 241G)	0	0
	beef broth or bouillon powder prep with water (1 CUP 244G)	2	0
	beef broth or boullion canned ready-to-serve (1 CUP 240G)	1	3

Food	Measure	X Risk-Points	✓ Life-Points
	chunky beef canned, ready-to-serve (1 CUP 240G)	19	12
	beef, mushroom, canned prep with eq vol water (1 CUP 244G)	11	4
	beef noodle, canned prep with eq vol water (1 CUP 244G)	8	5
	beef noodle dehydrated, prep with water (1 CUP 251G)	2	2
	chili beef canned prep with eq vol water (1 CUP 250G)	25	9
	consommé with gelatin dehydrated, prep with water (1 CUP 249G)	0	1
	oxtail dehydrated prep with water (1 CUP 253G)	9	2
	tomato beef with noodle, canned prep with eq vol water (1 CUP 244G)	11	5
	vegetable beef dehydrated, prep with water (1 CUP 253G)	4	3
	vegetable beef prep with eq vol water (1 CUP 244G)	6	6
SWEETBREADS	braised (3 OZ 85G)	54	12
T-BONE STEAK	choice, lean and fat, broiled (3 OZ 85G)	54	19
TENDERLOIN	choice, lean and fat, broiled (3 OZ 85G)	50	20
TONGUE	simmered (3 OZ 85G)	56	18

Food	Measure	X Risk-Points	✓ Life-Points
TOP ROUND	all grades, lean and fat, roasted (3 OZ 85G)	27	20

Chicken

Food	Measure	X Risk-Points	✓ Life-Points
BREADED AND FRIED	boneless pieces (6 PIECES 102G)	44	12
BREAST MEAT	with skin, fried in batter (1/2 BREAST 140G)	46	22
	with skin, roasted (1/2 BREAST 98G)	19	17
	without skin, roasted (1/2 BREAST 86G)	7	16
DRUMSTICKS	with skin, fried in batter (1 DRUMSTICK 72G)	28	9
	with skin, roasted (1 DRUMSTICK 52G)	14	7
	without skin, roasted (1 DRUMSTICK 44G)	6	6
FRANKFURTER	(1, 45G)	21	4
PASTE, LIVER	canned (1 OZ 28G)	9	18
ROASTER	light meat without skin, roasted (1 CUP 140G)	14	21
SALAD	with vegetables tossed without dressing (1½ CUPS 218G)	5	15
SANDWICH	fillet, plain (1 SANDWICH 182G)	73	19

Food	Measure	✗ Risk-Points	✓ Life-Points
	fillet, with cheese (1 SANDWICH 228G)	96	27
Soup	dehydrated broth or bouillion, prep with water (1 CUP 244G)	2	0
	canned broth, prep with eq vol water (1 CUP 244G)	3	4
	chunky canned, ready-to-serve (1 CUP 251G)	16	9
	cream of, canned, prep with eq vol water (1 CUP 244G)	18	3
	cream of, dehydrated, prep with water (1 CUP 261G)	25	7
	cream of, prep with eq vol milk (1 CUP 248G)	34	9
	gumbo, canned, prep with eq vol water (1 CUP 244G)	3	3
	chunky canned with meatballs, ready-to-serve (1 CUP 248G)	8	7
	canned with mushrooms, prep with eq vol water (1 CUP 244G)	22	4
	chunky canned with noodles, ready-to-serve (1 CUP 240G)	15	9
	with noodles, canned, prep with eq vol water (1 CUP 241G)	6	3
	with noodles, dehydrated, prep with water (1 CUP 252G)	2	2

Food	Measure	X Risk- Points	✓ Life- Points
	chunky canned with rice, ready-to-serve (1 CUP 240G)	7	9
	with rice, dehydrated, prep with water (1 CUP 253G)	3	1
	chunky canned with vegetables, ready-to-serve (1 CUP 240G)	12	10
	canned with vegetables, prep with eq vol water (1 CUP 241G)	7	4
	dehydrated with vegetables, prep with water (1 CUP 251G)	2	3
SPREAD	canned (1 OZ 28G)	8	2
THIGH	with skin, roasted (1 THIGH 62G)	24	8
WING	with skin, fried in batter (1 WING 49G)	26	5
	with skin, roasted (1 WING 34G)	16	4

Duck

Food	Measure	X Risk- Points	✓ Life- Points
DUCK	without skin, roasted (½ DUCK 221G)	69	37
	with skin, roasted (½ DUCK 382G)	277	45

Goose

Food	Measure	✗ Risk-Points	✓ Life-Points
GOOSE	without skin, roasted (½ GOOSE 591G)	202	**62**
	with skin, roasted (½ GOOSE 774G)	424	**60**
LIVER PATÉ	canned (paté de foie gras) smoked (1 OZ 28G)	31	**12**

Turkey

Food	Measure	✗ Risk-Points	✓ Life-Points
ALL TYPES	breast meat with skin, roasted (1 4 OZ SERVING 115G)	21	**17**
	breast meat without skin, roasted (2 SLICES 43G)	1	**8**
	breast (prebasted meat with skin), roasted (1 4 OZ SERVING 115G)	9	**15**
	canned meat without skin, with broth (1 4 OZ SERVING 115G)	19	**15**
	dark meat with skin, roasted (1 4 OZ SERVING 115G)	33	**17**
	diced light and dark meat without skin, seasoned (1 4 OZ SERVING 115G)	17	**12**

Food	Measure	Risk-Points	Life-Points
	leg meat with skin, roasted (1 4 OZ SERVING 115G)	28	17
	light meat, without skin, roasted (1 4 OZ SERVING 115G)	9	18
	wing meat with skin, roasted (1 WING 186G)	57	26
GROUND	(3 OZ 85G)	26	11
PATTIES	breaded, battered, fried (1 PATTY 2.25 OZ 64G)	28	6
ROAST BONELESS	frozen seasoned light and dark meat without skin, roasted (1 4 OZ SERVING 115G)	16	20
ROLL	light and dark meat (2 SLICES 57G)	9	6
	light meat (2 SLICES 57G)	10	7
SAUSAGE	bologna (2 SLICES 2 OZ 57G)	21	5
	pastrami (2 SLICES 2 OZ 57G)	8	6
	salami (2 SLICES 2 OZ 57G)	19	5
SOUP	chunky ready-to-serve (1 CUP 236G)	11	18
	noodle, canned prep with eq vol water (1 CUP 244G)	5	4
	vegetable, canned prep with eq vol water (1 CUP 241G)	7	4
STICKS	breaded, battered, fried (2 STICKS 5 OZ 128G)	54	12

Food	Measure	X Risk-Points	✓ Life-Points
THIGH	prebasted meat with skin, roasted (1 THIGH 314G)	67	**35**
WITH GRAVY	frozen (1 PKG 5 OZ 142G)	9	7

Gravy

Food	Measure	X Risk-Points	✓ Life-Points
AU JUS	canned (1 CUP 238G)	1	6
	dehydrated, prep with water (1 CUP 246G)	4	0
BEEF	canned (1 CUP 233G)	20	7
BROWN	dehydrated, prep with water (1 CUP 258G)	6	2
CHICKEN	canned (1 CUP 238G)	34	6
	dehydrated, prep with water (1 CUP 260G)	4	3
MUSHROOM	canned (1 CUP 238G)	16	6
	dehydrated, prep with water (1 CUP 258G)	3	3
ONION	dehydrated, prep with water (1 CUP 261G)	3	1
PORK	dehydrated, prep with water (1 CUP 258G)	5	3

Food	Measure	✗ Risk-Points	✓ Life-Points
TURKEY	canned (1 CUP 238G)	12	7
	dehydrated, prep with water (1 CUP 261G)	4	4

Lamb

Food	Measure	✗ Risk-Points	✓ Life-Points
GROUND	broiled (3 OZ 85G)	51	20
LEG	whole, lean and fat, roasted (3 OZ 85G)	43	20
LOIN	chop, lean and fat, broiled (3 OZ 85G)	62	20
	chop, lean and fat, roasted (3 OZ 85G)	65	19
RIB	chop, lean and fat, broiled (3 OZ 85G)	80	19
SCOTCH BROTH	canned, prep with eq vol water (1 CUP 241G)	8	5
SHANK	lean and fat, braised (3 OZ 85G)	35	21
SHOULDER	lean and fat, roasted (3 OZ 85G)	53	20
STEWING OR KABOBS	lean, braised (3 OZ 85G)	20	22
	lean, broiled (3 OZ 85G)	16	22

Pork

Food	Measure	✗ Risk-Points	✓ Life-Points
BACON	Canadian-style, grilled (2 SLICES 47G)	9	9
	streaky breakfast strips (3 SLICES 34G)	32	9
CENTER LOIN	chop, lean and fat, broiled (3 OZ 85G)	30	20
	chop, lean and fat, pan-fried (3 OZ 85G)	38	21
	lean and fat, roasted (3 OZ 85G)	32	17
CENTER RIB	chops, lean and fat, pan-fried (3 OZ 85G)	40	17
	chops, lean only, broiled (3 OZ 85G)	22	21
	chops, lean only, pan-fried (3 OZ 85G)	25	18
CORNDOG	hotdog with corn flour coating (1 CORNDOG 175G)	47	21
FEET	pickled (3 OZ 85G)	35	7
	simmered (3 OZ 85G)	27	5
HAM	and cheese loaf or roll (1 SLICE OR 1 OZ 28G)	15	4
	and cheese spread (1 OZ 28G)	18	4
	boneless extra lean (APPROX 5% FAT) roasted (3 OZ 85G)	11	16
	boneless regular (APPROX 11% FAT) roasted (3 OZ 85G)	19	17

Food	Measure	✗ Risk-Points	✓ Life-Points
	canned extra lean (APPROX 4% FAT) roasted (3 OZ 85G)	10	18
	patties grilled (1 PATTY 60G)	49	7
	salad spread (1 OZ 28G)	11	3
	whole, fully trimmed, roasted (3 OZ 85G)	11	17
HOTDOG	plain (1 HOTDOG 98G)	38	13
	with chili (1 HOTDOG 114G)	36	14
LEG	rump, half lean and fat, roasted (3 OZ 85G)	33	17
LUNCHEON MEAT	headcheese (1 SLICE OR 1 OZ 28G)	11	3
	olive loaf (1 SLICE OR 1 OZ 28G)	12	4
	pickle and pimiento loaf (1 SLICE OR 1 OZ 28G)	16	11
	pork and beef, i.e. Mortadella (1 SLICE OR 1 OZ 28G)	24	4
	pork, canned (1 OZ 28G)	22	3
SANDWICH	ham and cheese (1 SANDWICH 146G)	48	20
	ham, egg, and cheese (1 SANDWICH 143G)	55	24
	spread, pork and beef (1 OZ 28G)	12	2
SAUSAGE	bologna (1 SLICE OR 1 OZ 28G)	14	4
	bratwurst (1 OZ 28G)	19	4

Food	Measure	✗ Risk-Points	✓ Life-Points
	braunschweiger (1 oz 28g)	23	18
	liverwurst (1 oz 28g)	22	18
	pork and beef, smoked link (1 LINK 68G)	54	10
	pork links or sausage meat (1 oz 28g)	22	6
	salami (1 SLICE OR 1 OZ 28G)	25	9
SHOULDER	lean and fat, roasted (3 oz 85g)	50	16
SPARERIBS	lean and fat, braised (3 oz 85g)	70	19
TENDERLOIN	lean and fat, roasted (3 oz 85g)	13	18
	lean only, roasted (3 oz 85g)	10	19

Veal

Food	Measure	✗ Risk-Points	✓ Life-Points
GROUND	broiled (3 oz 85g)	19	17
LEG	cutlet, lean and fat, breaded and pan-fried (3 oz 85g)	19	19
	cutlet, lean only, breaded and pan-fried (3 oz 85g)	13	20
LOIN	chop, lean and fat braised (3 oz 85g)	42	17

Fish and Seafood

Food	Measure	✗ Risk-Points	✓ Life-Points
ABALONE	mixed species, fried (3 OZ 85G)	14	10
ANCHOVY	canned in oil (5 ANCHOVIES 20G)	4	5
BASS	freshwater mixed species, cooked dry heat (1 FILLET 62G)	7	11
	sea mixed species, cooked dry heat (1 FILLET 101G)	6	10
	striped, cooked dry heat (1 FILLET 124G)	9	19
BLUEFISH	cooked dry heat (1 FILLET 117G)	15	22
BUTTERFISH	cooked dry heat (1 FILLET 25G)	6	4
CARP	cooked dry heat (1 FILLET 170G)	30	25
CATFISH	channel, cooked breaded and fried (1 FILLET 87G)	28	13
	channel, cooked dry heat (1 FILLET 143G)	10	18
CAVIAR	black and red granular (1 TBSP 16G)	7	11
CLAM	chowder, canned Manhattan, chunky ready-to-serve (1 CUP 240G)	15	16
	chowder, canned Manhattan, with tomato without milk prep with eq vol wtr (1 CUP 244G)	5	12
	chowder, canned New England, with milk, prep with eq vol milk (1 CUP 248G)	22	16

Food	Measure	✗ Risk-Points	✓ Life-Points
	chowder, canned New England, with milk, prep with eq vol water (1 CUP 244G)	7	11
	mixed species, canned (3 OZ 85G)	4	27
	mixed species, cooked, breaded, and fried (3 OZ 85G)	23	20
	mixed species, cooked, moist heat (3 OZ 85G)	4	27
COD	Atlantic, canned (3 OZ 85G)	1	10
	Atlantic, cooked dry heat (1 FILLET 180G)	3	22
	Atlantic, dried and salted (3 OZ 85G)	5	29
	liver oil (1 TBSP 14G)	34	7
	Pacific, cooked dry heat (1 FILLET 90G)	1	11
CRAB	Alaska king, cooked moist heat (1 LEG 134G)	5	26
	Alaska king, imitation made from surimi (3 OZ 85G)	2	7
	baked (1 CRAB 109G)	5	29
	blue, canned (3 OZ 85G)	2	11
	blue, cooked moist heat (3 OZ 85G)	3	19
	blue, crab cakes (1 CAKE 60G)	11	15
	cake (1 CAKE 60G)	25	16

Food	Measure	Risk-Points ✗	Life-Points ✓
	queen, cooked moist heat (3 OZ 85G)	3	20
	soft-shell, fried (1 CRAB 125G)	44	15
	soup, canned ready-to-serve (1 CUP 244G)	3	7
CRAYFISH	mixed species, cooked moist heat (3 OZ 85G)	2	14
CUSK	cooked dry heat (1 FILLET 95G)	2	13
CUTTLEFISH	mixed species, cooked moist heat (3 OZ 85G)	2	31
EEL	mixed species, cooked dry heat (1 FILLET 159G)	59	28
FISH FILLET	battered or breaded and fried (1 FILLET 91G)	27	12
FISH SANDWICH	with tartar sauce (1 SANDWICH 158G)	56	17
	with tartar sauce and cheese (1 SANDWICH 183G)	71	21
FISH STICKS	frozen reheated (1 STICK 28G)	8	4
FLOUNDER/ SOLE	cooked dry heat (1 FILLET 127G)	4	18
GEFILTEFISH	(1 PIECE 42G)	1	3
GROUPER	mixed species, cooked dry heat (1 FILLET 202G)	6	21
HADDOCK	cooked dry heat (1 FILLET 150G)	3	23
	smoked (3 OZ 85G)	2	14

Food	Measure	✗ Risk-Points	✓ Life-Points
HALIBUT	Atlantic and Pacific, cooked dry heat (½ FILLET 159G)	11	28
	Greenland, cooked dry heat (½ FILLET 159G)	70	18
HERRING	Atlantic, cooked dry heat (1 FILLET 143G)	41	25
	Atlantic, kippered (1 FILLET 40G)	12	13
	Atlantic, pickled (1 PIECE 15G)	6	3
	oil (1 TBSP 14G)	34	0
	Pacific, cooked dry heat (1 FILLET 144G)	64	24
LOBSTER	northern, cooked moist heat (3 OZ 85G)	1	14
	spiny, mixed species, cooked moist heat (1 LOBSTER 163G)	7	30
MACKEREL	Atlantic, cooked dry heat (1 FILLET 88G)	39	20
	jack, canned (1 4 OZ SERVING 115G)	18	23
	king, cooked dry heat (½ FILLET 154G)	9	36
	Pacific and jack, mixed species, cooked dry heat (1 FILLET 176G)	44	35
MONKFISH	cooked dry heat (3 OZ 85G)	4	9
MULLET	striped, cooked dry heat (1 FILLET 93G)	11	12

Food	Measure	✗ Risk-Points	✓ Life-Points
MUSSEL	blue, cooked moist heat (3 OZ 85G)	9	24
OCEAN PERCH	Atlantic, cooked dry heat (1 FILLET 50G)	2	7
OCTOPUS	cooked moist heat (3 OZ 85G)	4	24
OYSTER	eastern, canned (3 OZ 85G)	5	22
	eastern, breaded and fried (6 MEDIUM OYSTERS 88G)	27	24
	eastern, cooked dry heat (6 MEDIUM OYSTERS 59G)	3	20
	Pacific, cooked moist heat (1 MEDIUM OYSTER 25G)	2	16
	stew, canned prepared with eq vol milk (1 CUP 245G)	37	20
	stew, canned prepared with eq vol water (1 CUP 241G)	18	16
PERCH	mixed species, cooked dry heat (1 FILLET 46G)	1	8
PIKE	northern, cooked dry heat (½ FILLET 155G)	3	22
	walleye, cooked dry heat (1 FILLET 124G)	4	23
POLLOCK	Atlantic, cooked dry heat (½ FILLET 151G)	4	23
	walleye, cooked dry heat (1 FILLET 60G)	1	11

Food	Measure	X Risk-Points	✓ Life-Points
POMPANO	Florida, cooked dry heat (1 FILLET 88G)	29	16
ROCKFISH	Pacific, mixed species, cooked dry heat (1 FILLET 149G)	7	20
ROE	mixed species, cooked dry heat (3 OZ 85G)	17	25
ROUGHY, ORANGE	cooked dry heat (3 OZ 85G)	1	15
SABLEFISH	cooked dry heat (½ FILLET 151G)	74	24
	smoked (3 OZ 85G)	42	16
SALMON	Atlantic farmed, cooked dry heat (½ FILLET 178G)	54	36
	Atlantic wild, cooked dry heat (½ FILLET 154G)	31	39
	Chinook, cooked dry heat (½ FILLET 154G)	51	31
	Chinook, smoked (lox) (3 OZ 85G)	9	14
	chum, canned (3 OZ 85G)	11	19
	chum, cooked dry heat (½ FILLET 154G)	18	28
	coho, cooked dry heat (1 FILLET 143G)	29	26
	oil (1 TBSP 14G)	34	0
	pink, canned (3 OZ 85G)	12	18

Food	Measure	✗ Risk-Points	✓ Life-Points
	pink, cooked dry heat (½ FILLET 124G)	13	23
	sockeye, canned (3 OZ 85G)	15	11
	sockeye, cooked dry heat (½ FILLET 155G)	42	26
SARDINE	Atlantic, canned in oil (2 SARDINES 24G)	6	11
	oil (1 TBSP 14G)	34	0
SCALLOP	mixed species, breaded and fried (2 LARGE SCALLOPS 31G)	8	3
	mixed species, imitation made from surimi (3 OZ 85G)	0	7
SEA TROUT	mixed species, cooked dry heat (1 FILLET 186G)	21	26
SHAD	American, cooked dry heat (1 FILLET 144G)	63	24
SHARK	mixed species, batter-dipped and fried (3 OZ 85G)	29	11
SHRIMP	breaded and fried (6–8 SHRIMP 164G)	62	16
	breaded and fried (4 LARGE SHRIMP 30G)	9	5
	canned (3 OZ 85G)	4	11
	cooked moist heat (4 LARGE SHRIMP 22G)	0	3
	imitation made from surimi (3 OZ 85G)	3	8

Food	Measure	✗ Risk-Points	✓ Life-Points
	soup, cream of, canned prep with eq vol milk (1 CUP 248G)	43	12
	soup, cream of, canned prep with eq vol water (1 CUP 244G)	24	4
SMELT	rainbow, cooked dry heat (3 OZ 85G)	6	15
SNAPPER	mixed species, cooked dry heat (1 FILLET 170G)	7	21
SQUID	mixed species, fried (3 OZ 85G)	15	12
STURGEON	mixed species, cooked dry heat (3 OZ 85G)	11	18
	mixed species, smoked (3 OZ 85G)	9	20
SUNFISH	pumpkinseed, cooked dry heat (1 FILLET 37G)	0	7
	pumpkinseed raw (1 FILLET 48G)	0	7
SURIMI	(3 OZ 85G)	1	8
SWORDFISH	cooked dry heat (1 PIECE 106G)	13	23
TILEFISH (TILAPIA)	cooked dry heat (½ FILLET 150G)	17	23
TROUT	mixed species, cooked dry heat (1 FILLET 62G)	13	17
	rainbow farmed, cooked dry heat (1 FILLET 71G)	12	17
	rainbow wild, cooked dry heat (1 FILLET 143G)	20	25

Food	Measure	✗ Risk-Points	✓ Life-Points
TUNA	fresh bluefin, cooked dry heat (3 OZ 85G)	13	24
	light meat, canned in oil (3 OZ 85G)	17	19
	light meat, canned in water (3 OZ 85G)	1	20
	salad (3 OZ 85G)	19	11
	salad submarine sandwich (1 SUB 256G)	69	29
	fresh skipjack, cooked dry heat (1/2 FILLET 154G)	4	34
	white meat canned in oil (3 OZ 85G)	17	18
	white meat canned in water (3 OZ 85G)	5	15
	fresh yellowfin, cooked dry heat (3 OZ 85G)	2	19
TURBOT	European, cooked dry heat (1/2 FILLET 159G)	15	20
WHITEFISH	mixed species, cooked dry heat (1 FILLET 154G)	28	23
	mixed species, smoked (3 OZ 85G)	1	15
WHITING	mixed species, cooked dry heat (1 FILLET 72G)	3	13
YELLOWTAIL	mixed species, cooked dry heat (1/2 FILLET 146G)	24	25

Butter

Food	Measure	✗ Risk-Points	✓ Life-Points
LIGHT	(1 TSP 5G)	10	0
OIL	anhydrous (1 CUP 205G)	951	4
	(1 TBSP 13G)	59	0
SALTED	(1 PAT 5G)	18	0
	(1 STICK 113G)	429	3
UNSALTED	(1 PAT 5G)	18	0
	(1 STK 4 OZ 113G)	429	3
WHIPPED	(1 PAT 4G)	14	0
	(1 STK 4 OZ 76G)	286	2

Cheese

Food	Measure	✗ Risk-Points	✓ Life-Points
BLUE CHEESE	(1 OZ 28G)	39	5
BRICK CHEESE	(1 OZ 28G)	39	5
BRIE	(1 OZ 28G)	36	6
CAMEMBERT	(1 OZ 28G)	32	6
CARAWAY CHEESE	(1 OZ 28G)	39	5

Food	Measure	✗ Risk-Points	✓ Life-Points
CHEDDAR	American domestic (1 OZ 28G)	44	5
	Cheddar-type, reduced fat (1 OZ 28G)	19	7
CHEESE FONDUE	(1 SERVING 80G)	77	13
CHEESE FOOD	cold pack American (1 OZ 28G)	32	5
CHEESE SOUFFLÉ	(1 CUP 136G)	86	17
CHEESE SPREAD	pasteurized processed (1 OZ 28G)	27	4
CHESHIRE	(1 OZ 28G)	40	5
COLBY	(1 OZ 28G)	42	5
COTTAGE CHEESE	creamed large or small curd (1 OZ 28G)	6	2
	creamed with fruit (1 OZ 28G)	4	1
	lowfat 1% fat (1 OZ 28G)	1	2
	lowfat 2% fat (1 OZ 28G)	2	2
	uncreamed dry large or small curd (1 OZ 28G)	0	2
CREAM CHEESE	(1 OZ 28G)	46	2
EDAM	(1 OZ 28G)	36	6
	Edam-type, reduced fat (1 OZ 28G)	14	1
FETA	(1 OZ 28G)	31	7
FONTINA	(1 OZ 28G)	40	5
FROMAGE FRĀIS	plain (1 OZ 28G)	9	3

Food	Measure	✗ Risk-Points	✓ Life-Points
	very low fat (1 OZ 28G)	0	3
GOAT CHEESE	hard type (1 OZ 28G)	52	8
	semisoft type (1 OZ 28G)	43	4
	soft type (1 OZ 28G)	30	4
GOUDA	(1 OZ 28G)	36	6
GRUYERE	(1 OZ 28G)	39	7
LIMBURGER	(1 OZ 28G)	35	5
MONTEREY JACK	(1 OZ 28G)	40	5
MOZZARELLA	part skim milk (1 OZ 28G)	21	5
	part skim milk low moisture (1 OZ 28G)	22	5
	whole milk (1 OZ 28G)	27	4
	whole milk low moisture (1 OZ 28G)	32	4
MUENSTER	(1 OZ 28G)	40	6
NEUFCHATEL	(1 OZ 28G)	31	1
PARMESAN	grated (1 OZ 28G)	40	8
	grated (1 TBSP 5G)	7	1
	piece (1 OZ 28G)	34	7
	shredded (1 TBSP 5G)	6	1
PORTSALUT	(1 OZ 28G)	35	5

Food	Measure	✗ Risk-Points	✓ Life-Points
PROCESSED CHEESE	American pasteurized (1 OZ 28G)	41	4
	pimiento pasteurized (1 OZ 28G)	41	5
	Swiss pasteurized (1 OZ 28G)	33	5
PROVOLONE	(1 OZ 28G)	35	6
QUICHE	cheese and mushroom (1 4 OZ SERVING 115G)	66	14
	Lorraine (1 4 OZ SERVING 115G)	107	15
RICOTTA	part skim milk (1 OZ 28G)	10	2
	whole milk (1 OZ 28G)	17	2
ROMANO	(1 OZ 28G)	35	7
ROQUEFORT	(1 OZ 28G)	40	6
SAUSAGE	cheesefurter cheese smokie (1 CHEESEFURTER 43G)	33	7
SOUP	canned condensed (1 CUP 257G)	100	9
	canned prep with eq vol milk (1 CUP 251G)	68	10
	canned prep with eq vol water (1 CUP 247G)	50	4
STILTON	blue (1 OZ 28G)	47	5
	white (1 OZ 28G)	41	4
SWISS	domestic (1 OZ 28G)	37	7
TILSIT	whole milk (1 OZ 28G)	35	7

Food	Measure	✗ Risk-Points	✓ Life-Points
WELSH RAREBIT	(1 SERVING 60G)	62	8

Cream

Food	Measure	✗ Risk-Points	✓ Life-Points
HALF & HALF	cream and milk (1 TBSP 15G)	8	0
	cream and milk (½ CUP 121G)	64	5
HEAVY WHIPPING	(1 TBSP 15G)	25	0
	(½ CUP OR 1 CUP WHIPPED 119G)	205	4
LIGHT COFFEE OR TABLE	(1 TBSP 15G)	13	0
	(½ CUP 120G)	108	5
LIGHT WHIPPING	(1 TBSP 15G)	21	0
	(½ CUP OR 1 CUP WHIPPED 120G)	174	4
MEDIUM	25% fat (1 TBSP 15G)	17	0
	25% fat (½ CUP 120G)	140	4
SOUR	(1 TBSP 12G)	11	0
	(½ CUP 115G)	112	5
	half & half cultured (1 TBSP 15G)	8	0
	half & half cultured (½ CUP 110G)	61	5

Food	Measure	X Risk-Points	✓ Life-Points
SUBSTITUTE	nondairy, with hydr veg oil and soy protein (1 TBSP 15G)	3	0
	nondairy, with hydr veg oil and soy protein (½ CUP 120G)	29	0
	nondairy, with lauric acid oil and sodium caseinate (1 TBSP 15G)	10	0
	nondairy, with lauric acid oil and sodium caseinate (½ CUP 120G)	83	0
WHIPPED	topping pressurized (1 TBSP 3G)	3	0
	topping pressurized (½ CUP 30G)	31	1

Eggs

Food	Measure	X Risk-Points	✓ Life-Points
CHICKEN EGG, WHITE ONLY	dried flakes or powder (1 OZ 28G)	0	9
	raw, fresh and frozen (1 LRG EGG WHITE 33G)	0	1
	raw, fresh and frozen (1 OZ 28G)	0	1
CHICKEN EGG, WHOLE	dried (1 OZ 28G)	29	18
	fried (1 LRG EGG 46G)	17	6
	hard-boiled (1 LRG EGG 50G)	13	7
	poached (LRG EGG 50G)	12	6

Food	Measure	X Risk-Points	✓ Life-Points
	raw, fresh and frozen (1 LRG EGG 50G)	12	7
CHICKEN EGG, YOLK ONLY	dried (1 OZ 28G)	43	19
	raw fresh (1 LRG EGG YOLK 17G)	12	5
DUCK EGG, WHOLE	fresh raw (1 EGG 70G)	24	18
EGG CUSTARD	baked prep from recipe (½ CUP 141G)	24	8
	dry mix prep with 2% milk (½ CUP 133G)	14	9
	dry mix prep with whole milk (½ CUP 133G)	22	8
EGG FRIED RICE	(1 4 OZ SERVING 115G)	30	5
EGG FU YUNG	(1 4 OZ SERVING 115G)	59	17
EGG ROLL	from Chinese restaurant (1 4 OZ SERVING 115G)	35	3
EGG SUBSTITUTE	frozen (1 OZ 28G)	7	2
	liquid (1 OZ 28G)	2	2
	powder (1 OZ 28G)	9	13
EGGNOG	(½ CUP 127G)	42	7
GOOSE EGG, WHOLE	fresh raw (1 EGG 144G)	47	28
OMELET	cheese (1 4 OZ SERVING 115G)	105	20

Food	Measure	✗ Risk-Points	✓ Life-Points
	plain (1 4 OZ SERVING 115G)	63	17
	Spanish (1 4 OZ SERVING 115G)	23	11
PANCAKES	blueberry (4″ PANCAKE 38G)	8	3
	buckwheat (4″ PANCAKE 30G)	5	3
	buttermilk (4″ PANCAKE 38G)	8	3
	plain (4″ PANCAKE 38G)	9	3
	pancakes with butter and syrup (3 CAKES 232G)	43	15
QUAIL EGG, WHOLE	fresh raw (1 EGG 9G)	2	1
QUICHE	Lorraine (1 4 OZ SERVING 115G)	107	15
	mushroom (1 4 OZ SERVING 115G)	75	12
SANDWICH	egg and cheese (1 SANDWICH 146G)	49	20
SCRAMBLED EGGS	(2 EGGS 94G)	43	16
TURKEY EGG, WHOLE	fresh raw (1 EGG 79G)	23	16

Milk

Food	Measure	✗ Risk-Points	✓ Life-Points
BUTTERMILK	dried (1 OZ 28G)	7	14

Food	Measure	✗ Risk-Points	✓ Life-Points
	fluid cultured from skim milk (1 CUP 245G)	10	10
CHOCOLATE DRINK	made with low-fat 1% fat milk (1 CUP 250G)	11	13
	made with whole milk (1 CUP 250G)	39	13
CHOCOLATE MILK	drink made with low-fat 2% fat milk (1 CUP 250G)	23	13
CONDENSED MILK	sweetened canned (1 FL OZ 38G)	15	4
EVAPORATED MILK	skimmed, canned (1 FL OZ 32G)	10	2
GOAT'S MILK	fluid (1 CUP 244G)	48	9
HOT COCOA	homemade chocolate beverage (1 CUP 250G)	42	14
ICE CREAM	chocolate (½ CUP 66G)	33	4
	French vanilla soft-serve (½ CUP 86G)	48	5
	strawberry (½ CUP 66G)	13	4
	sundae caramel (1 SUNDAE 155G)	33	9
	sundae hot fudge (1 SUNDAE 158G)	37	10
	sundae strawberry (1 SUNDAE 153G)	28	9
	vanilla (½ CUP 66G)	33	4
	vanilla, rich (½ CUP 74G)	55	4
ICE MILK	vanilla (½ CUP 66G)	13	5

Food	Measure	✗ Risk-Points	✓ Life-Points
	vanilla soft-serve (½ CUP 88G)	10	5
	vanilla soft-serve with cone (1 CONE 103G)	26	6
LOW-FAT MILK	fluid pasteurized and raw 1% fat (1 CUP 244G)	12	12
	fluid pasteurized and raw 2% fat (1 CUP 245G)	21	13
MALTED MILK	beverage (1 CUP MILK PLUS ¾ OZ PWD 265G)	44	17
	chocolate flavor beverage (1 CUP MILK PLUS ¾ OZ PWD 265G)	41	14
MILKSHAKE	thick chocolate (1 CONTAINER 10.6 OZ 300G)	37	16
	thick vanilla (1 CONTAINER 11 OZ 313G)	44	19
SKIMMED MILK	fluid pasteurized and raw fluid (protein fortified with added vitamin A) (1 CUP 246G)	2	15
WHOLE MILK	dried (1 OZ 28G)	35	11
	fluid low-sodium pasteurized and raw (1 CUP 244G)	39	10
	fluid pasteurized and raw 3.3% fat (1 CUP 244G)	38	12
	fluid pasteurized and raw 3.7% fat (1 CUP 244G)	41	12

Yogurt

Food	Measure	Risk-Points ✗	Life-Points ✓
CHOCOLATE	frozen, soft-serve (1 CUP 144G)	39	9
LOW-FAT	coffee and vanilla 11 gm protein per 8 oz (1 CONTAINER 8 OZ NT WT 227G)	13	16
	fruit 10 grams protein per 8 oz (1 CONTAINER 8 OZ NT WT 227G)	11	14
	fruit 11 grams protein per 8 oz (1 CONTAINER 8 OZ NT WT 227G)	15	16
	fruit 9 grams protein per 8 oz (1 CONTAINER 8 OZ NT WT 227G)	12	13
	plain 12 grams protein per 8 oz (1 CONTAINER 8 OZ NT WT 227G)	17	17
SKIM MILK	plain 13 grams protein per 8 oz (1 CONTAINER 8 OZ NT WT 227G)	1	19
VANILLA	soft-serve (1 CUP 144G)	36	8
WHOLE MILK	plain 8 grams protein per 8 oz (1 CONTAINER 8 OZ NT WT 227G)	35	11

LifePoints Food Group Six:
Drinks, Desserts, Snacks, and Sauces

Drinks

Note that many other drinks are also listed in food groups one and three.

Drink	Measure	✗ Risk-Points	✓ Life-Points
BLOODY MARY	1 cocktail (5 FL OZ 148G)	0	3
BOURBON AND SODA	1 cocktail (4 FL OZ 116G)	0	0
CAROB FLAVOR BEVERAGE	mix prepared from powder with milk (1 CUP MILK PLUS 3 TSP PWD 256G)	38	12
CHOCOLATE FLAVOR BEVERAGE	mix prepared from powder with milk (1 CUP MILK PLUS 3 TSP PWD 266G)	41	13
CITRUS FRUIT JUICE DRINK	frozen concentrate prepared with water (1 CUP 248G)	0	3
COFFEE	brewed, made with single cream (6 FL OZ CUP 190G)	9	1
	brewed, made with whole milk (6 FL OZ CUP 190G)	4	1
	brewed, made with semiskimmed milk (6 FL OZ CUP 190G)	1	1
	cappuccino made with cream and chocolate (1 CUP 212G)	33	1

Food	Measure	Risk-Points	Life-Points
	instant, cappuccino flavor prepared with water (6 FL OZ WTR PLUS 2 RD TSP 192G)	13	0
	instant, French flavor prepared with water (6 FL OZ WTR PLUS 2 RD TSP 189G)	22	0
	instant, mocha flavor prepared with water (6 FL OZ WTR PLUS 2 RD TSP 188G)	12	0
CRANBERRY JUICE COCKTAIL	(6 FL OZ 187G)	0	0
DAIQUIRI	1 cocktail (2 FL OZ 60G)	0	0
EGGNOG	prepared with milk from powder (1 CUP MILK PLUS 3 TSP PWD 272G)	38	12
FRUIT PUNCH DRINK	canned (6 FL OZ 186G)	0	1
GIN AND TONIC	1 cocktail (7.5 OZ 225G)	0	0
LEMONADE FLAVOR DRINK	powder prepared with water (1 CUP WATER PLUS 2 TBSP PWD 266G)	0	0
	frozen concentrate, prepared with water (1 CUP 248G)	0	1
LIMEADE	Frozen concentrate, prepared with water (1 CUP 247G)	0	0
MANHATTAN	1 cocktail (2 FL OZ 57G)	0	0
MARTINI	1 cocktail (2.5 OZ 70G)	0	0

Food	Measure	X Risk-Points	✓ Life-Points
ORANGE DRINK	breakfast type with juice and pulp prep with water from frozen (6 FL OZ 188G)	0	16
ORANGE FLAVOR DRINK	breakfast type prepared with water (6 FL OZ 186G)	0	8
	Gelatin-based prepared with water from powder (4 FL OZ WATER PLUS 1 PKT 136G)	0	1
PINA COLADA	1 cocktail (4.5 OZ 141G)	9	2
SCREWDRIVER	1 cocktail (7 FL OZ 213G)	0	6
STRAWBERRY FLAVOR BEVERAGE	powder prepared with milk (1 CUP MILK PLUS 3 TSP PWD 266G)	38	12
TEA	brewed (1 CUP 230G)	0	0
	instant (1 CUP WATER PLUS 3 TSP PWD 259G)	0	1
TEQUILA SUNRISE	1 cocktail (5.5 OZ 172G)	0	3
TOM COLLINS	1 cocktail (7.5 OZ 222G)	0	0
WHISKEY SOUR	1 cocktail (3 FL OZ 90G)	0	2

Biscuits and Cookies

Food	Measure	✗ Risk-Points	✓ Life-Points
BISCUITS	mixed grain refrigerated dough baked (1 BISCUIT 41G)	6	4
	plain or buttermilk commercially baked (1 BISCUIT 35G)	14	3
	plain or buttermilk dry mix prepared (1 BISCUIT 57G)	17	6
	plain or buttermilk (1 BISCUIT 60G)	24	7
	plain or buttermilk refrigerated dough higher fat baked (1 BISCUIT 27G)	9	2
	plain or buttermilk refrigerated dough lower fat baked (1 BISCUIT 21G)	2	2
	with egg (1 BISCUIT 136G)	50	15
	with egg and bacon (1 BISCUIT 150G)	77	17
	with egg and ham (1 BISCUIT 192G)	67	26
	with egg and sausage (1 BISCUIT 180G)	112	24
	with egg and steak (1 BISCUIT 148G)	71	23
	with egg, cheese, and bacon (1 BISCUIT 144G)	85	19
	with ham (1 BISCUIT 113G)	85	14
	with sausage (1 BISCUIT 124G)	106	14

Food	Measure	✗ Risk-Points	✓ Life-Points
	with steak (1 BISCUIT 141G)	64	18
COOKIES	animal crackers (INCLUDES ARROWROOT TEA) (1 OZ 28G)	9	2
	brownies commercially prepared (1 OZ 28G)	11	2
	brownies dry mix regular prepared (1 OZ 28G)	14	1
	brownies dry mix special dietary prepared (1 OZ 28G)	10	1
	brownies (1 OZ 28G)	20	2
	butter commercially prepared enriched (1 OZ 28G)	22	3
	butter commercially prepared unenriched (1 OZ 28G)	22	1
	chocolate chip commercially prepared regular higher fat enriched (1 OZ 28G)	16	2
	chocolate chip commercially prepared regular higher fat unenriched (1 OZ 28G)	16	1
	chocolate chip commercially prepared regular lower fat (1 OZ 28G)	10	2
	chocolate chip commercially prepared soft type (1 OZ 28G)	17	1
	chocolate chip commercially prepared special dietary (1 OZ 28G)	17	2

Food	Measure	X Risk-Points	✓ Life-Points
	chocolate chip dry mix prepared (1 OZ 28G)	18	2
	chocolate chip made with butter (1 OZ 28G)	29	2
	chocolate chip made with margarine (1 OZ 28G)	20	2
	chocolate chip refrigerated dough baked (1 OZ 28G)	16	1
	chocolate sandwich with creme filling regular (1 OZ 28G)	14	2
	chocolate sandwich with creme filling regular chocolate-coated (1 OZ 28G)	18	1
	chocolate sandwich with extra creme filling (1 OZ 28G)	17	1
	chocolate wafers (1 OZ 28G)	10	2
	coconut macaroons (1 OZ 28G)	23	0
	fig bars (1 OZ 28G)	5	2
	fortune cookies (1 OZ 28G)	1	1
	gingersnaps (1 OZ 28G)	6	3
	graham crackers chocolate-coated (1 OZ 28G)	22	2
	graham crackers plain or honey (includes cinnamon) (1 OZ 28G)	7	3
	ladyfingers with lemon juice and rind (1 OZ 28G)	6	4

Food	Measure	Risk-Points	Life-Points
	ladyfingers without lemon juice and rind (1 OZ 28G)	6	4
	marshmallow chocolate-coated (includes marshmallow pies) (1 OZ 28G)	11	1
	molasses (1 OZ 28G)	9	3
	oatmeal commercially prepared regular (1 OZ 28G)	12	2
	oatmeal commercially prepared soft-type (1 OZ 28G)	10	2
	oatmeal dry mix prepared (1 OZ 28G)	13	2
	oatmeal with raisins (1 OZ 28G)	11	2
	oatmeal without raisins (1 OZ 28G)	12	2
	oatmeal refrigerated dough baked (1 OZ 28G)	14	1
	peanut butter commercially prepared regular (1 OZ 28G)	16	2
	peanut butter commercially prepared soft-type (1 OZ 28G)	17	1
	prepared soft-type (1 OZ 28G)	17	1
	peanut butter (1 OZ 28G)	16	2
	peanut butter refrigerated dough baked (1 OZ 28G)	19	2
	peanut butter sandwich regular (1 OZ 28G)	14	3

Food	Measure	✗ Risk-Points	✓ Life-Points
	raisin soft-type (1 OZ 28G)	9	2
	shortbread commercially prepared pecan (1 OZ 28G)	23	2
	shortbread commercially prepared plain (1 OZ 28G)	17	2
	shortbread made with butter (1 OZ 28G)	43	2
	shortbread made with margarine (1 OZ 28G)	23	2
	sugar commercially prepared regular (includes vanilla) (1 OZ 28G)	14	2
	sugar commercially prepared special dietary (1 OZ 28G)	9	2
	sugar made with butter (1 OZ 28G)	30	2
	sugar made with margarine (1 OZ 28G)	16	2
	sugar refrigerated dough baked (1 OZ 28G)	16	1
	sugar wafers with creme filling regular (1 OZ 28G)	17	1
	vanilla sandwich with creme filling (1 OZ 28G)	14	2
	vanilla wafers higher fat (1 OZ 28G)	13	2
	vanilla wafers lower fat (1 OZ 28G)	10	2

Cakes, Pastries, and Puddings

Food	Measure	✗ Risk-Points	✓ Life-Points
CAKE	angelfood (1 OZ 28G)	0	2
	Boston cream pie (1 OZ 28G)	6	1
	carrot prepared without frosting (1 OZ 28G)	11	3
	carrot with cream cheese frosting (1 OZ 28G)	18	1
	cheesecake (1 OZ 28G)	24	1
	cheesecake with cherry topping (1 OZ 28G)	21	1
	cherry fudge with chocolate frosting (1 OZ 28G)	8	1
	chocolate with chocolate frosting (1 OZ 28G)	11	1
	chocolate without frosting (1 OZ 28G)	8	2
	coffeecake, cheese (1 OZ 28G)	10	2
	coffeecake, cinnamon with crumb topping (1 OZ 28G)	16	2
	coffeecake, creme-filled with chocolate frosting (1 OZ 28G)	7	1
	coffeecake, fruit (1 OZ 28G)	7	2
	cupcakes, creme-filled chocolate with frosting (1 CUPCAKE 50G)	18	4

Food	Measure	✗ Risk-Points	✓ Life-Points
	cupcakes, creme-filled sponge (1 CUPCAKE 43G)	12	2
	fruitcake (1 OZ 28G)	6	1
	German chocolate with coconut-nut frosting (1 OZ 28G)	13	1
	gingerbread (1 OZ 28G)	11	2
	marble without frosting (1 OZ 28G)	12	1
	pineapple upside-down (1 OZ 28G)	8	1
	pound, made with margarine (1 OZ 28G)	11	2
	pound, prepared with butter (1 OZ 28G)	23	1
	shortbiscuit-type (1 SHORTCAKE 65G)	23	6
	sponge (1 OZ 28G)	1	2
	white, with coconut frosting (1 OZ 28G)	8	1
	white, without frosting (1 OZ 28G)	10	1
	yellow, with chocolate frosting (1 OZ 28G)	12	1
	yellow, with vanilla frosting (1 OZ 28G)	10	1
	yellow, without frosting (1 OZ 28G)	11	1
CREAM PUFFS	shell only (1 CREAM PUFF SHELL 66G)	42	7
	shell with custard filling (1 CREAM PUFF 130G)	50	11

Food	Measure	✗ Risk-Points	✓ Life-Points
CROUTONS	plain (1 CUP 30G)	4	4
	seasoned (1 CUP 40G)	18	6
DANISH PASTRY	cheese (1 PASTRY 91G)	61	9
	cinnamon (1 PASTRY 88G)	41	8
	fruit (1 PASTRY 94G)	39	8
	lemon (1 PASTRY 71G)	32	3
	nut (includes almond raisin nut cinnamon nut) (1 PASTRY 65G)	40	6
	raspberry (1 PASTRY 71G)	32	3
DOUGHNUTS	cake-type, chocolate, sugared or glazed (1 MED DOUGHNUT 42G)	20	3
	cake-type, plain, (includes unsugared old-fashioned) (1 MED DOUGHNUT 47G)	26	3
	cake-type, plain, chocolate-coated or frosted (1 MED DOUGHNUT 43G)	33	3
	cake-type, plain, sugared or glazed (1 MED DOUGHNUT 45G)	25	3
	French crullers glazed (1 CRULLER 41G)	18	2
	honey buns (1 MED DOUGHNUT 60G)	34	6
	raised, with creme filling (1 DOUGHNUT 85G)	52	7
	raised, with jelly filling (1 DOUGHNUT 86G)	39	6

Food	Measure	✗ Risk-Points	✓ Life-Points
ÉCLAIRS	custard-filled with chocolate glaze (1 ÉCLAIR 100G)	39	8
FLAN	caramel custard (1 OZ 28G)	4	1
ICE CREAM CONES	cake or wafer-type (1 CONE 4G)	0	0
	sugar rolled-type (1 CONE 10G)	0	1
PASTRY	phyllo dough (1 SHEET DOUGH 19G)	2	2
	puff frozen ready-to-bake baked (1 SHELL 40G)	38	3
PIE	apple (1 OZ 28G)	7	0
	apple strudel (1 STRUDEL 71G)	19	2
	banana cream (1 OZ 28G)	14	1
	blueberry (1 OZ 28G)	7	0
	butterscotch pudding-type (1 OZ 28G)	10	2
	cherry (1 OZ 28G)	7	0
	chocolate cream (1 OZ 28G)	11	2
	chocolate mousse (1 OZ 28G)	17	1
	coconut cream (1 OZ 28G)	21	1
	coconut custard (1 OZ 28G)	12	1
	egg custard (1 OZ 28G)	6	1
	filling, canned apple (1 OZ 28G)	0	0
	filling, canned cherry (1 OZ 28G)	0	0

Food	Measure	✗ Risk-Points	✓ Life-Points
	fried cherry (1 FRIED 128G)	51	6
	fried fruit (1 FRIED 128G)	51	6
	fried lemon (1 FRIED 128G)	51	6
	lemon meringue (1 OZ 28G)	6	1
	mince (1 OZ 28G)	7	1
	peach (1 OZ 28G)	7	0
	pecan (1 OZ 28G)	13	1
	pumpkin (1 OZ 28G)	6	2
	vanilla cream (1 OZ 28G)	10	2
POPOVERS	made with whole milk (1 POPOVER 40G)	8	4
PUDDING	banana dry mix instant prep with 2% milk (½ CUP 147G)	11	6
	banana dry mix instant prep with whole milk (½ CUP 147G)	19	6
	banana dry mix regular prep with 2% milk (½ CUP 140G)	11	6
	banana dry mix regular prep with whole milk (½ CUP 140G)	19	5
	banana ready-to-eat (½ CUP 126G)	11	4
	bread (½ CUP 126G)	21	7
	chocolate dry mix instant prep with 2% milk (½ CUP 147G)	12	6

Food	Measure	Risk-Points	Life-Points
	chocolate dry mix instant prep with whole milk (½ CUP 147G)	20	7
	chocolate dry mix regular prep with 2% milk (½ CUP 142G)	13	6
	chocolate dry mix regular prep with whole milk (½ CUP 142G)	22	6
	chocolate prep with 2% milk (½ CUP 157G)	14	6
	chocolate prep with whole milk (½ CUP 157G)	23	6
	chocolate ready-to-eat (½ CUP 157G)	15	5
	coconut cream dry mix inst prep with whole milk (½ CUP 147G)	23	6
	coconut cream dry mix instant prep with 2% milk (½ CUP 147G)	15	6
	coconut cream dry mix reg prep with whole milk (½ CUP 140G)	26	6
	coconut cream dry mix regular prep with 2% milk (½ CUP 140G)	18	7
	lemon dry mix instant prep with 2% milk (½ CUP 147G)	11	6
	lemon dry mix instant prep with whole milk (½ CUP 147G)	19	6
	lemon ready-to-eat (½ CUP 146G)	10	0
	rice dry mix prep with 2% milk (½ CUP 144G)	10	7

Food	Measure	X Risk-Points	✓ Life-Points
	rice dry mix prep with whole milk (1/2 CUP 144G)	19	6
	rice (1/2 CUP 152G)	19	7
	rice ready-to-eat (1/2 CUP 144G)	27	4
	tapioca dry mix prep with 2% milk (1/2 CUP 141G)	10	6
	tapioca dry mix prep with whole milk (1/2 CUP 141G)	19	5
	tapioca (1/2 CUP 152G)	24	9
	tapioca ready-to-eat (1/2 CUP 152G)	14	5
	vanilla dry mix instant prep with 2% milk (1/2 CUP 142G)	10	6
	vanilla dry mix instant prep with whole milk (1/2 CUP 142G)	18	6
	vanilla dry mix regular prep with 2% milk (1/2 CUP 140G)	11	6
	vanilla dry mix regular prep with whole milk (1/2 CUP 140G)	19	5
	vanilla (1/2 CUP 123G)	19	5
	vanilla ready-to-eat (1/2 CUP 123G)	11	3
TOASTER PASTRIES	brown sugar-cinnamon (1 TOASTER PASTRY 50G)	17	9
	fruit (includes apple, blueberry, cherry, strawberry) (1 TOASTER PASTRY 52G)	13	8

Dressings and Sauces

Food	Measure	✗ Risk-Points	✓ Life-Points
CATSUP	(1 TBSP 15G)	0	0
COLESLAW	(½ CUP 60G)	16	2
CREAM SUBSTITUTE	nondairy, powdered (½ CUP 46G)	112	1
	nondairy, powdered (1 TSP 2G)	4	0
DESSERT TOPPING	nondairy, prepared from powder (1 TBSP 4G)	3	0
	nondairy pressurized (1 TBSP 4G)	5	0
	nondairy semisolid frozen (1 TBSP 4G)	6	0
FROSTINGS	chocolate creamy prep with butter (1 OZ 28G)	15	0
	chocolate creamy prep with margarine (1 OZ 28G)	8	0
	chocolate creamy ready-to-eat (1 OZ 28G)	12	0
	coconut-nut ready-to-eat (1 OZ 28G)	17	0
	cream cheese–flavor ready-to-eat (1 OZ 28G)	12	0
	glaze (1 OZ 28G)	5	0
	seven minute (1 OZ 28G)	0	0
	sour cream–flavor ready-to-eat (1 OZ 28G)	12	0

Food	Measure	Risk-Points	Life-Points
	vanilla creamy prep with butter (1 OZ 28G)	5	0
	vanilla creamy prep with margarine (1 OZ 28G)	7	0
	vanilla creamy ready-to-eat (1 OZ 28G)	11	0
PICKLE	cucumber dill (1 MEDIUM 65G)	0	0
	cucumber sour (1 MEDIUM 35G)	0	0
	cucumber sweet (1 MEDIUM 35G)	0	0
	relish, hamburger (1 TBSP 15G)	0	0
	relish, hot dog (1 TBSP 15G)	0	0
	relish, sweet (1 TBSP 15G)	0	0
SALAD DRESSING	blue plus Roquefort cheese regular (1 TBSP 15G)	20	0
	French low-fat 5 cal/tsp (1 TBSP 16G)	2	0
	French regular (1 TBSP 16G)	15	0
	Italian low-fat 2 cal/tsp (1 TBSP 15G)	3	0
	Italian regular (1 TBSP 15G)	17	0
	mayonnaise, eggless, soybean (1 TBSP 15G)	7	0
	mayonnaise, regular, soybean (1 TBSP 14G)	27	0
	Russian low-fat (1 TBSP 16G)	1	0

Food	Measure	X Risk-Points	✓ Life-Points
	sesame seed (1 TBSP 15G)	17	0
	thousand island low-fat 10 cal/tsp (1 TBSP 15G)	4	0
	thousand island regular (1 TBSP 16G)	13	0
	vinegar and oil (1 TBSP 16G)	19	0
SAUCE	barbecue sauce (½ CUP 125G)	5	3
	bearnaise dehydrated prep with milk and butter (½ CUP 127G)	156	5
	cheese dehydrated prep with milk (½ CUP 140G)	35	9
	curry dehydrated prep with milk (½ CUP 136G)	22	8
	hollandaise with butterfat, dehydrated prep with water (½ CUP 130G)	43	5
	hollandaise with veg oil dehydrated, prep with milk and butter (½ CUP 127G)	156	5
	marinara canned (½ CUP 125G)	10	5
	mushroom dehydrated prep with milk (½ CUP 133G)	20	10
	sour cream dehydrated prep with milk (½ CUP 157G)	60	10
	soy made from hydrolyzed vegetable protein (1 TBSP 18G)	0	0
	soy, wheat-free (tamari) (1 TBSP 18G)	0	1

Food	Measure	X Risk-Points	✓ Life-Points
	canned spaghetti (½ CUP 125G)	14	7
	stroganoff dehydrated prep with milk and water (½ CUP 148G)	25	11
	sweet and sour dehydrated prep with water and vinegar (½ CUP 157G)	0	2
	teriyaki dehydrated prep with water (½ CUP 142G)	1	3
	teriyaki ready-to-serve (1 TBSP 18G)	0	0
	white dehydrated prep with milk (½ CUP 132G)	24	7
SOUR CREAM, IMITATION	nondairy cultured (1 OZ 28G)	37	0
SYRUPS	chocolate fudge-type (1 TBSP 21G)	8	1
	corn, dark (1 TBSP 20G)	0	0
	corn, light (1 TBSP 20G)	0	0
	malt (1 TBSP 24G)	0	2
	maple (1 TBSP 20G)	0	0
	sorghum (1 TBSP 21G)	0	1
	table blends all types (1 TBSP 20G)	0	0
TOPPINGS	butterscotch or caramel (1 TBSP 20G)	0	0
	marshmallow cream (1 OZ 28G)	0	0
	nuts in syrup (1 TBSP 20G)	11	1
	pineapple (1 TBSP 20G)	0	0

Food	Measure	✗ Risk-Points	✓ Life-Points
	strawberry (1 TBSP 20G)	0	0
VINEGAR	all types (1 TBSP 15G)	0	0

Snacks and Sweets

Food	Measure	✗ Risk-Points	✓ Life-Points
CANDIES	butterscotch (1 PIECE 6G)	0	0
	caramels (1 PIECE 8G)	3	0
	caramels chocolate-flavor roll (1 PIECE 6G)	0	0
	carob (1 BAR 3 OZ 87G)	71	17
	chewing gum (1 STICK 3G)	0	0
	divinity (1 PIECE 11G)	0	0
	fondant (1 PIECE 16G)	0	0
	fudge brown sugar with nuts (1 PIECE 14G)	3	0
	fudge chocolate marshmallow (1 PIECE 20G)	15	0
	fudge chocolate marshmallow with nuts (1 PIECE 22G)	16	0
	fudge chocolate (1 PIECE 17G)	6	0
	fudge chocolate with nuts (1 PIECE 19G)	8	0

Food	Measure	✗ Risk-Points	✓ Life-Points
	fudge peanut butter (1 PIECE 16G)	2	0
	fudge vanilla (1 PIECE 16G)	4	0
	fudge vanilla with nuts (1 PIECE 15G)	4	0
	gumdrops (starch jelly pieces) (10 SMALL 35G)	0	0
	jellybeans (10 SM 11G)	0	0
	marshmallows (1 REGULAR 7G)	0	0
	peanut brittle (1 OZ 28G)	13	3
	praline (1 PIECE 39G)	23	2
	sesame crunch (1 OZ 28G)	23	7
	taffy (1 PIECE 15G)	2	0
	toffee (1 PIECE 12G)	18	0
	truffles (1 PIECE 12G)	19	0
CHOCOLATES	baking chocolate liquid (1 PACKET 1 OZ 28G)	53	2
	baking chocolate squares (1 OZ 28G)	69	3
	dark sweet chocolate bar (1 BAR 1.45 OZ 41G)	30	2
	milk chocolate (1 BAR 1.55 OZ 44G)	60	4
	milk chocolate coated peanuts (10 PIECES 40G)	43	5
	milk chocolate coated raisins (10 PIECES 10G)	6	0

Food	Measure	X Risk-Points	✓ Life-Points
	milk chocolate with almonds (1 BAR 1.45 OZ 41G)	52	5
	milk chocolate with rice cereal (1 BAR 1.4 OZ 40G)	47	3
	semisweet chocolate (1 OZ APPROX 60 PCS 28G)	37	1
	semisweet chocolate made with butter (1 OZ APPROX 60 PCS 28G)	37	1
	sweet chocolate (1 BAR 1.45 OZ 41G)	61	2
	sweet chocolate coated fondant (1 SM PATTY 11G)	4	0
FAST FOODS	burrito with beans (2 BURRITOS 217G)	51	28
	burrito with beans and cheese (2 BURRITOS 186G)	51	23
	burrito with beans and chile peppers (2 BURRITOS 204G)	57	29
	burrito with beans and meat (2 BURRITOS 231G)	62	33
	burrito with beans, cheese, and beef (2 BURRITOS 203G)	53	24
	burrito with beans, cheese, and chile peppers (2 BURRITOS 336G)	83	48
	burrito with beef (2 BURRITOS 220G)	78	32
	burrito with beef and chile peppers (2 BURRITOS 201G)	59	27

Food	Measure	Risk-Points	Life-Points
	burrito with beef, cheese, and chile peppers (2 BURRITOS 304G)	77	46
	burrito with fruit (apple or cherry) (1 SMALL BURRITO 74G)	34	7
	enchilada with cheese (1 ENCHILADA 163G)	79	17
	enchilada with cheese and beef (1 ENCHILADA 192G)	67	24
	frijoles with cheese (1 CUP 167G)	30	19
	nachos with cheese (6–8 NACHOS 113G)	58	15
	nachos with cheese and jalapeño peppers (6–8 NACHOS 204G)	105	24
	nachos with cheese, beans, ground beef, and peppers (6–8 NACHOS 255G)	93	26
	nachos with cinnamon and sugar (6–8 NACHOS 109G)	136	17
	taco (1 SMALL TACO 171G)	85	21
	taco salad (1½ CUPS 198G)	51	16
	taco salad with chili con carne (1½ CUPS 261G)	45	22
	taco shells baked (1 MED 13G)	7	1
	taco shells baked without added salt (1 MED 13G)	7	1

Food	Measure	✗ Risk-Points	✓ Life-Points
	tortillas ready-to-bake or fry, corn (1 MED 25G)	1	2
	tortillas ready-to-bake or fry, flour (1 MED 35G)	6	4
	tostada with beans and cheese (1 TOSTADA 144G)	40	16
	tostada with beans, beef, and cheese (1 TOSTADA 225G)	86	23
	tostada with beef and cheese (1 TOSTADA 163G)	77	21
	tostada with guacamole (1 TOSTADA 130G)	36	12
	wonton wrappers (includes egg roll wrappers) (1 WONTON WRAPPER 8G)	0	1
FROZEN DESSERTS	fruit and juice bars (1 BAR 2.5 FL OZ 77G)	0	0
	gelatin pops (1 POP 44G)	0	0
	ice pops (1 BAR 1.75 FL OZ 52G)	0	0
	ices, water, and fruit (4 FL OZ 96G)	0	0
	ices, water, pineapple, coconut (4 FL OZ 96G)	6	2
	pudding pops, chocolate (1 POP 47G)	5	2
	pudding pops, vanilla (1 POP 47G)	5	2
	sherbet, orange (1 BAR 2.75 FL OZ 66G)	5	1

Food	Measure	✗ Risk-Points	✓ Life-Points
FRUIT BUTTERS	apple (1 TBSP 18G)	0	0
HONEY	(1 TBSP 21G)	0	0
JAMS AND PRESERVES	(1 TBSP 20G)	0	0
JELLIES	(1 TBSP 19G)	0	0
MARMALADE	orange (1 TBSP 20G)	0	0
MOLASSES	(1 TBSP 20G)	0	1
	Blackstrap (1 TBSP 20G)	0	4
SHERBET	orange (8 FL OZ 193G)	17	4
SNACKS	banana chips (1 OZ 28G)	61	1
	corn cakes (1 CAKE 9G)	0	0
	corn-based extruded chips, barbecue flavor (1 OZ 28G)	23	2
	corn-based extruded chips, plain (1 OZ 28G)	23	2
	corn-based extruded cones, nacho flavor (1 OZ 28G)	56	1
	corn-based extruded cones, plain (1 OZ 28G)	48	2
	corn-based extruded cones, onion flavor (1 OZ 28G)	16	3
	corn-based extruded puffs or twists, cheese flavor (1 OZ 28G)	24	4

Food	Measure	Risk-Points	Life-Points
	corn-based extruded puffs or twists, cheese-flavor enriched (1 OZ 28G)	24	3
	crisped rice bar, almond (1 OZ BAR 28G)	14	12
	crisped rice bar, chocolate chip (1 OZ BAR 28G)	11	7
	fruit leather bars (1 BAR 23G)	6	0
	fruit leather bars with cream (1 BAR 24G)	4	0
	fruit leather pieces (1 OZ 28G)	5	1
	fruit leather rolls (1 LG ROLL 21G)	1	0
	granola bars, hard almond (1 BAR 24G)	22	1
	granola bars, hard chocolate chip (1 BAR 24G)	20	2
	granola bars, hard peanut (1 BAR 24G)	12	2
	granola bars, hard peanut butter (1 BAR 24G)	14	1
	granola bars, hard plain (1 BAR 25G)	12	2
	granola bars, soft-coated milk chocolate coating chocolate chip (1.25 OZ BAR 35G)	37	3

Food	Measure	✗ Risk-Points	✓ Life-Points
	granola bars, soft-coated milk chocolate coating peanut butter (1 BAR 37G)	46	3
	granola bars, soft uncoated chocolate chip (1.5 OZ BAR 43G)	32	4
	granola bars, soft uncoated chocolate chip graham and marshmallow (1 OZ BAR 28G)	19	2
	granola bars, soft uncoated nut and raisin (1 OZ BAR 28G)	20	3
	granola bars, soft uncoated peanut butter (1 OZ BAR 28G)	11	3
	granola bars, soft uncoated peanut butter and chocolate chip (1 OZ BAR 28G)	14	3
	granola bars, soft uncoated plain (1 OZ BAR 28G)	15	3
	granola bars, soft uncoated raisin (1.5 OZ DAR 43G)	30	4
	meat-based sticks, smoked (1 STICK 20G)	30	3
	oriental mix, rice-based (1 OZ 28G)	37	6
	popcorn, air-popped (1 OZ 28G)	2	4
	popcorn, air-popped white popcorn (1 OZ 28G)	2	3
	popcorn cakes (1 CAKE 10G)	0	1

Food	Measure	X Risk-Points	✓ Life-Points
	popcorn, caramel-coated with peanuts (1 OZ 28G)	5	2
	popcorn, caramel-coated without peanuts (1 OZ 28G)	9	1
	popcorn, cheese-flavor (1 OZ 28G)	23	3
	popcorn, oil-popped (1 OZ 28G)	19	3
	popcorn, oil-popped white popcorn (1 OZ 28G)	19	2
	potato chips, light (1 OZ 28G)	14	3
	potato chips, plain (1 OZ 28G)	27	2
	potato sticks (1 OZ 28G)	24	3
	pretzels, hard confectioner's coating chocolate-flavor (1 PRETZEL 11G)	6	0
	pretzels, hard plain (10 TWISTS 60G)	5	11
	sesame sticks, wheat-based (1 OZ 28G)	26	2
	taro chips (10 CHIPS 23G)	14	1
	tortilla chips, light (1 OZ 28G)	10	2
	tortilla chips, plain (1 OZ 28G)	18	2
	trail mix, regular (1 OZ 28G)	20	5
	trail mix with chocolate chips, salted nuts, and seeds (1 OZ 28G)	22	5
	trail mix, tropical (1 OZ 28G)	18	3

Food	Measure	✗ Risk-Points	✓ Life-Points
SUGAR	brown (1 OZ 28G)	0	0
	granulated (1 OZ 28G)	0	0
	maple (1 OZ 28G)	0	1
	powdered (1 OZ 28G)	0	0

Margarines, Oils, and Spreads

Food	Measure	✗ Risk-Points	✓ Life-Points
MARGARINE	blended 60% corn oil and 40% butter (1 TSP 5G)	10	0
	imitation, approximately 40% fat (1 TSP 5G)	4	0
	regular, hard, made with coconut oil (hydrogenated) (1 TSP 5G)	20	0
	regular, hard, made with oils other than coconut (hydrogenated) (1 TSP 5G)	9	0
	soft, unspecified oils (1 TSP 5G)	9	0
MARGARINELIKE SPREAD	approximately 60% fat stick or tub (hydrogenated) (1 TSP 5G)	7	0
OIL	almond (1 TBSP 14G)	34	0
	apricot kernel (1 TBSP 14G)	34	0
	avocado (1 TBSP 14G)	35	0

Food	Measure	✗ Risk-Points	✓ Life-Points
	canola (1 TBSP 14G)	35	0
	cocoa butter (1 TBSP 14G)	60	0
	coconut (1 TBSP 14G)	88	0
	corn, salad or cooking (1 TBSP 14G)	34	0
	cottonseed, salad or cooking (1 TBSP 14G)	34	0
	hazelnut (1 TBSP 14G)	34	0
	mustard (1 TBSP 14G)	35	0
	nutmeg butter (1 TBSP 14G)	91	0
	oat (1 TBSP 14G)	34	0
	olive, salad or cooking (1 TBSP 14G)	33	0
	palm (1 TBSP 14G)	50	0
	palm kernel (1 TBSP 14G)	83	0
	peanut, salad or cooking (1 TBSP 14G)	33	0
	poppyseed (1 TBSP 14G)	34	0
	rice bran (1 TBSP 14G)	34	0
	safflower, salad or cooking linoleic (over 70%) (1 TBSP 14G)	34	0
	safflower, salad or cooking oleic (over 70%) (1 TBSP 14G)	34	0
	sesame, salad or cooking (1 TBSP 14G)	34	0

Food	Measure	✗ Risk-Points	✓ Life-Points
	soybean, lecithin (1 TBSP 14G)	34	0
	soybean, salad or cooking (1 TBSP 14G)	34	0
	soybean, salad or cooking (hydrogenated) (1 TBSP 14G)	34	0
	soybean, salad or cooking (hydrogenated) and cottonseed (1 TBSP 14G)	34	0
	sunflower, linoleic (60% and over) (1 TBSP 14G)	34	0
	sunflower, linoleic (hydrogenated) (1 TBSP 14G)	34	0
	sunflower, linoleic (less than 60%) (1 TBSP 14G)	34	0
	sunflower, oleic (70% and over) (1 TBSP 14G)	35	0
	walnut (1 TBSP 14G)	34	0
	wheat germ (1 TBSP 14G)	34	0
SANDWICH SPREAD	with chopped pickle and regular unspecified oils (1 TBSP 15G)	13	0
SHORTENING	household and mutipurpose; for baking, bread, and frostings (1 TBSP 13G)	32	0
	frying, with beef tallow (1 TBSP 13G)	43	0
	frying, with palm (1 TBSP 13G)	45	0
	frying, regular (1 TBSP 13G)	32	0

Food	Measure	✗ Risk-Points	✓ Life-Points
	household, lard and vegetable oil (1 TBSP 13G)	38	0

Herbs and Spices

Food	Measure	✗ Risk-Points	✓ Life-Points
ALLSPICE	ground (1 TBSP 6G)	1	1
ANISE	seed (1 TBSP 7G)	2	2
BASIL	fresh (2 TBSP 5G)	0	0
	ground (1 TBSP 5G)	0	2
BAY LEAF	crumbled (1 TBSP 2G)	0	0
CARAWAY	seed (1 TBSP 7G)	2	2
CARDAMOM	ground (1 TBSP 6G)	0	1
CELERY	seed (1 TBSP 7G)	4	3
CHERVIL	dried (1 TBSP 2G)	0	0
CHILI	powder (1 TBSP 8G)	3	2
CINNAMON	ground (1 TBSP 7G)	0	3
CLOVES	ground (1 TBSP 7G)	3	1
CORIANDER	leaf, dried (1 TBSP 2G)	0	1
	raw (9 PLANTS 20G)	0	1
	seed (1 TBSP 5G)	2	1

Food	Measure	Risk-Points	Life-Points
CUMIN	seed (1 TBSP 6G)	3	3
CURRY	powder (1 TBSP 6G)	2	2
DILL	seed (1 TBSP 7G)	2	2
	weed, dried (1 TBSP 3G)	0	1
	weed, fresh (1 CUP SPRIGS 9G)	0	1
FENNEL	seed (1 TBSP 6G)	2	1
FENUGREEK	seed (1 TBSP 11G)	1	3
GARLIC	powder (1 TBSP 8G)	0	0
GINGER	ground (1 TBSP 5G)	0	0
MACE	ground (1 TBSP 5G)	4	1
MARJORAM	dried (1 TBSP 2G)	0	1
MUSTARD	seed, yellow (1 TBSP 11G)	8	3
NUTMEG	ground (1 TBSP 7G)	13	0
ONION	powder (1 TBSP 7G)	0	0
OREGANO	ground (1 TBSP 5G)	1	2
PAPRIKA	(1 TBSP 7G)	2	4
PARSLEY	dried (1 TBSP 1G)	0	1
PEPPER	black (1 TBSP 6G)	0	1
	red or cayenne (1 TBSP 5G)	2	1
	white (1 TBSP 7G)	0	0
POPPY	seed (1 TBSP 9G)	9	3

Food	Measure	✗ Risk-Points	✓ Life-Points
POULTRY SEASONING	(1 TBSP 4G)	0	1
PUMPKIN PIE SPICE	(1 TBSP 6G)	1	1
ROSEMARY	dried (1 TBSP 3G)	1	1
SAFFRON	(1 TBSP 2G)	0	0
SAGE	ground (1 TBSP 2G)	1	0
SAVORY	ground (1 TBSP 4G)	0	2
SESAME	seeds dry decorticated (1 TBSP 8G)	10	2
TARRAGON	ground (1 TBSP 5G)	0	2
THYME	ground (1 TBSP 4G)	0	4
TURMERIC	ground (1 TBSP 7G)	1	2

NOTES

1. D. B. Allison, et al., "Counting Calories—Caveat Emptor," *Journal of the American Medical Association* 270 (September 22–29, 1993): 1454–6.

2. R. J. Kuczmarski, et al., "Increasing Prevalence of Overweight Among US Adults: The National Health and Nutrition Examination Surveys, 1960 to 1991," *JAMA* 272 (July 20, 1994): 205–7.

3. S. W. Lichtman, et al., "Discrepancy Between Self-reported and Actual Caloric Intake and Exercise in Obese Subjects," *New England Journal of Medicine* 327 (December 31, 1992): 1893–8.

4. The Associated Press, December 31, 1992.

5. *Time* 145 (January 16, 1995).

6. S. B. Eaton, et al., *The Paleolithic Prescription* (New York: Harper & Row, 1988).

7. M. A. Rookus, et al., "Changes in Body Mass Index in Young Adults in Relation to Number of Life Events Experienced," *International Journal of Obesity* 12 (1988): 29–39.

8. "Diet and Health: Implications for Reducing

Chronic Disease Risk," Committee on Diet and Health of the National Research Council: Washington D.C.: National Academy Council, 1989.

9. UPI, January 6, 1990.

10. Beta-Carotene. American Hospital Formulary Service, February, 1987. American Society of Hospital Pharmacists, Inc.

11. *Science* 264 (April 22, 1994).

12. D. Harman, *Proceedings of the National Academy of Science* 88 (1991): 5360–5363.

13. "In Search of Methuselah: Estimating the Upper Limits to Human Longevity." *Science* 250 (November 2, 1990): 634–640.

14. D. Harman, 5360–5363.

15. D. Harman, "Free Radical Theory of Aging." *Free Radicals: From Basic Science To Medicine*. Poli G. Albano and E. Dianzani MU, eds. (Basel: Birkhauser Verlag, 1993).

16. Media statement, Alliance for Aging Research, March 3, 1994.

17. Anonymous, "The Effect of Vitamin E and Beta-Carotene on the Incidence of Lung Cancer and Other Cancers in Male Smokers," *N Engl J Med* 330 (April 14, 1994): 1029–35.

18. "Beta-Carotene: Helpful or Harmful?" *Science* 264 (April 22, 1994): 500–501.

19. C. H. Hennekens, et al., "Lack of Effect of Long-term Supplementation with Beta-Carotene on the Incidence of Malignant Neoplasms and Cardiovascular Disease," *N Engl J Med* 334 (May 2, 1996): 1145–9.

20. D. K. Pandey, et al., "Dietary Vitamin C and

Beta-Carotene and Risk of Death in Middle-aged Men," *American Journal of Epidemiology* 142 (December 15, 1995): 1269–78.

21. "Vitamin C Exhibits Remarkable Antioxidant Powers," *Better Nutrition* 51 (December, 1989): 10.

22. M. A. Helser, et al., "Influence of Fruit and Vegetable Juices on the Endogenous Formation of N-Nitrosoproline and N-Nitrosothiazolidine-4-Carboxylic Acid in Humans on Controlled Diets," *Carcinogenesis* 13 (December, 1992): 2277–80.

23. J. VanEenwyk, et al., "Folate, Vitamin C, and Cervical Intraepithelial Neoplasia." *Cancer Epidemiol Biomarkers Prev* 1 (2) (January–February 1992): 119–124.

24. J. Chen, et al., *Diet, Life-style and Mortality in China. A Study of the Characteristics of 65 Counties*, (Oxford University Press, Cornell University Press, and the China People's Medical Publishing House, 1990).

25. L. K. Mahan and M. T. Arlin, eds. *Krause's Food Nutrition and Diet Therapy*. W. B. Saunders Company, 1992.

26. Y. Schutz, J. P. Flatt, and E. Jequier, "Failure of Dietary Fat Intake to Promote Fat Oxidation: A Factor Favoring the Development of Obesity," *American Journal of Clinical Nutrition* 50 (1989): 307–14.

27. L. J. Beilin, "Strategies and Difficulties in Dietary Intervention in Myocardial Infarction Patients," *Clinical and Experimental Hypertension* 14 (1992): 213.

28. *New York Times,* May 8, 1990.

29. A. Barbeau, M. Roy, G. Bernier, G. Campanella, and S. Paris, "Ecogenetics of Parkinson's Disease: Prevalence and Environmental Aspects in Rural Areas," *Canadian Journal of Neurological Science* 14 (February, 1987): 36–41.

30. W. C. Willett, "Diet and Health: What Should We Eat?" *Science* 264 (April 22, 1994): 532–537.

31. D. A. Snowdon, et al., "Meat Consumption and Fatal Ischemic Heart Disease," *Preventive Medicine* 13 (September, 1984): 490–500.

32. T. Hirayama, "Mortality in Japanese with Lifestyles Similar to Seventh-Day Adventists: Strategy for Risk Reduction by Life-style Modification," *National Cancer Institute Monograph* 69 (December, 1985): 143–53.

33. M. Thorogood, et al., "Risk of Death from Cancer and Ischaemic Heart Disease in Meat and Nonmeat Eaters," *British Medical Journal* 308 (June 25, 1994): 667–70.

34. CNN, September 17, 1996.

35. Barnard, Neal, *Food for Life* (New York: Harmony Books, 1993).

36. A. Kendall, et al., *Am J Clin Nutr* 53 (1991): 1124–29.

37. *Tufts University Diet and Nutrition Letter* 13 (May, 1995): 4.

38. Ibid.

39. Ibid.

40. H. Otto, et al., *Diatetik bei Diabetes Mellitus* (Berne: Verlag hans Huber, 1973), 41–50.

41. J. Yetiv, *Popular Nutritional Practices: A Scientific Appraisal,* (Popular Medicine Press, 1986).

42. T. M. S. Wolever, et al., *Am J Clin Nutr* 54 (1991): 846–54.

43. D. L. Trout, et al., *Am J Clin Nutr* 58 (1993): 873–78.

44. Wolever, *op. cit.*

45. D. J. Jenkins, et al., *N Engl J Med* 14 (1989): 929–34.

INDEX

Page numbers in **boldface** refer to the LifePoints Counter.